AF333181

PSYCHOTROPIC MEDICATION FOR CHILDREN IN FOSTER CARE

OVERSIGHT AND GUIDANCE ISSUES

PSYCHIATRY - THEORY, APPLICATIONS AND TREATMENTS

Additional books in this series can be found on Nova's website
under the Series tab.

Additional e-books in this series can be found on Nova's website
under the eBooks tab.

PSYCHOTROPIC MEDICATION FOR CHILDREN IN FOSTER CARE

OVERSIGHT AND GUIDANCE ISSUES

MALCOLM C. BURGESS

EDITOR

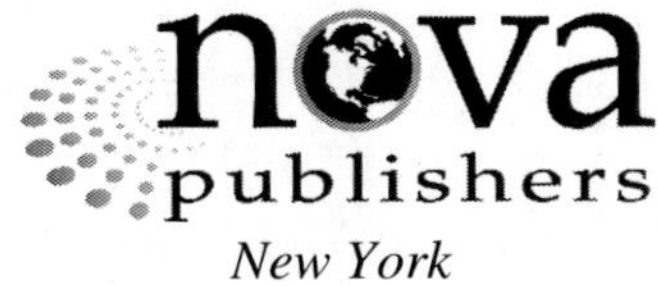

nova publishers

New York

NOTICE TO THE READER

Library of Congress Cataloging-in-Publication Data

ISBN: 978-1-63485-155-8

Published by Nova Science Publishers, Inc. † New York

CONTENTS

PREFACE

Children in foster care are children that the state has removed from their homes and placed in another setting designed to provide round-the-clock care (e.g., foster family home, group home, child care institution). The large majority of children enter foster care because of neglect or abuse at the hands of their parents. Maltreatment by a caregiver is often traumatic for children, and may lead to children having challenges regulating their emotions and interpreting cues and communication from others, among other problem behaviors. Children in foster care are more likely to have mental health care needs than children generally. Children in foster care who have mental health needs may receive psychosocial services such as individual or group counseling and case management to improve their health. Alternatively, or in addition, a medical professional may prescribe psychotropic medications. These are prescribed drugs that affect the brain chemicals related to mood and behavior. They are used to treat a variety of mental health conditions including attention disorders, depression, anxiety, conduct disorders, and others. While psychotropic medication alone is not necessarily advised, children in foster care may more readily receive psychotropics to treat their mental health needs due to the complexity of their symptoms and the lack of appropriate screening and assessment and/or the limited availability of health care professionals trained to provide effective therapies (e.g., cognitive behavioral therapy). This book discusses psychotropic medication for children in foster care. It also provides additional federal guidance which could help states better plan for oversight of psychotropic medications administered by managed-care organizations.

In: Psychotropic Medication …
Editor: Malcolm C. Burgess

ISBN: 978-1-63485-155-8
© 2016 Nova Science Publishers, Inc.

Chapter 1

CHILD WELFARE: OVERSIGHT OF PSYCHOTROPIC MEDICATION FOR CHILDREN IN FOSTER CARE[*]

Adrienne L. Fernandes-Alcantara,
Sarah W. Caldwell and Emilie Stoltzfus

SUMMARY

Children in foster care are children that the state has removed from their homes and placed in another setting designed to provide round-the-clock care (e.g., foster family home, group home, child care institution). The large majority of children enter foster care because of neglect or abuse at the hands of their parents. Maltreatment by a caregiver is often traumatic for children, and may lead to children having challenges regulating their emotions and interpreting cues and communication from others, among other problem behaviors. Children in foster care are more likely to have mental health care needs than children generally.

Children in foster care who have mental health needs may receive psychosocial services such as individual or group counseling and case management to improve their health. Alternatively, or in addition, a medical professional may prescribe psychotropic medications. These are prescribed drugs that affect the brain chemicals related to mood and behavior. They are used to treat a variety of mental health conditions

---

[*] This is an edited, reformatted and augmented version of a Congressional Research Service, Publication No. R43466, dated July 28, 2015.

including attention disorders, depression, anxiety, conduct disorders, and others. While psychotropic medication alone is not necessarily advised, children in foster care may more readily receive psychotropics to treat their mental health needs due to the complexity of their symptoms and the lack of appropriate screening and assessment and/or the limited availability of health care professionals trained to provide effective therapies (e.g., cognitive behavioral therapy).

Between 16% and 33% of children in out-of-home care may be using psychotropic medication on any given day, although the rate of use varies significantly based on certain factors, including the child's age, placement setting, and length of involvement with the child welfare agency. Among children generally, about 6% are taking psychotropic medications (at some point during a given year). Some of the difference in prevalence of use may be explained by the higher levels of mental health risk factors among children in foster care.

The use of psychotropics by children in foster care has come under increased scrutiny by policymakers and stakeholders in the child welfare field. Little research has been conducted to show whether psychotropics are effective and safe for children who need mental health services. Despite these concerns, some children may benefit from specific psychotropic medication for managing mental and behavioral symptoms associated with their exposure to traumatic events. The President's FY2016 budget proposes a five-year initiative to reduce reliance on psychotropic medications for children in foster care by encouraging the use of evidence-based screening, assessment, and treatment of trauma and mental health disorders. Congress has also taken a strong interest in oversight of prescription medications used by children in care, addressing the issue in oversight hearings and other fact-finding forums. Further, federal law (Title IV-B, Subpart 1 of the Social Security Act) requires states to describe their oversight of prescription medications for children in foster care, including specific protocols used with regard to psychotropic medication.

The Congressional Research Service (CRS) reviewed state plans submitted to HHS in 2012 that described state protocols in five areas identified by HHS as important to monitoring and appropriate use of psychotropic medication. States' responses were wide ranging, and oversight efforts are nascent in some states and fairly robust in others. With regard to screening for mental health need and planning treatment: Mental health evaluations appear to be available for children generally who are entering care, though some states limit this kind of evaluation to children of a minimum age (e.g., age three or older). States most frequently indicated that evaluations are conducted, within 30 days of removal from the home, by a primary care physician or a mental health professional such as a psychiatrist. With regard to consent and assent for the use of psychotropic medications by children in care, and methods for ongoing communication between stakeholders involved in the child's health care: Over half of states that responded reported that a parent or legal guardian is involved in providing consent. With regard to effective medication monitoring at both the client and agency level: States reported that monitoring at the child (i.e., client) level is primarily focused on determining how the medication is affecting the child and may be carried out by a foster caregiver, caseworker, and or clinician. Agency monitoring, which tracks use of psychotropics at a system level, may be conducted by the child welfare agency, an overall health program for children in foster care, or special committees or review boards.

The findings from the state plans suggest policy issues that may be relevant to Congress as it considers the next steps in oversight of psychotropic use among children in foster care. These issues include possible broader use of medical homes and electronic health records to improve oversight of psychotropic medications, the role of Medicaid in improving screenings and services for children in care with mental health needs, the involvement of youth in choosing their mental health care, and the extent to which states should report to HHS on their oversight policies.

INTRODUCTION

Children in foster care are more likely to have mental health care needs than children generally. They are also more likely than other children to receive psychotropic medications, which are prescribed drugs that affect the brain chemicals related to mood and behavior.[1] Psychotropic medications are used to treat a variety of mental health conditions including attention disorders, depression, anxiety, conduct disorders, and others. On the one hand, prescription of psychotropic medication for foster children may be appropriate, given their mental health needs. Still, the evidence on the safety and efficacy of psychotropics in children is limited. Congress has taken a strong interest in how states are monitoring and regulating use of these medications. Federal child welfare law requires states to have a plan for overseeing prescription drug use among children in foster care, including the use of psychotropic medications.

This report first provides background on the mental health needs of children in foster care, and the prevalence of psychotropic medication use among these children. The next section of the report discusses congressional oversight of psychotropic medication, and recent efforts taken by the U.S. Department of Health and Human Services (HHS) to provide assistance to states in ensuring appropriate use of psychotropic medications for children in care and to fund an initiative that would encourage states to implement evidence-based psychosocial interventions as an alternative to prescribing psychotropic medications. Following this is a discussion of current federal requirements concerning state monitoring of the use of these medications for foster children. The final section of the report includes a review by the Congressional Research Service (CRS) of plans submitted by states to HHS that address oversight of psychotropic and other prescription medications. The report concludes with a brief discussion of policy implications in light of the findings from the CRS review.

CHILDREN IN FOSTER CARE

Children in foster care are children that the state has removed from their homes and placed in another setting that is designed to provide round-the-clock care (e.g., foster family home, group home, child care institution). Placement in foster care means that a judge has determined that the child's removal from his or her home was necessary because the home was "contrary to the welfare" of the child and, accordingly, the judge has given responsibility for the child's "care and placement" to the state child welfare agency.[2] Most children enter foster care because of neglect or abuse experienced at the hands of their parents, although a child's behavior problem may also be a factor in foster care placement. This is especially true for children entering care at an older age.[3] Foster care is intended to be a temporary placement until a child can be reunited with his or her parent(s), or when this is not possible, until a permanent placement with relatives, an adopted family, or a legal guardian can be found. While working to find them permanent homes, states must attend to the safety and well-being of children in foster care, including their physical and mental health.

During FY2013, some 641,000 children spent at least one day (24 hours) in foster care and 238,000 left the system, resulting in more than 402,000 of those children remaining in care on the last day of that fiscal year. Although there is variation at the state level, the national foster care caseload has generally been in decline for more than a decade. Across the nation, there were 122,000 fewer children in foster care on the last day of FY2013 as compared to the last day of FY2002 (when 524,000 were in care).[4]

MENTAL HEALTH NEEDS OF CHILDREN IN FOSTER CARE

Children in foster care have higher mental health service needs than children generally.[5] The abuse or neglect children experience before entering foster care can have serious mental health outcomes. Maltreatment by a parent or other caregiver is stressful for children and may alter how their brains develop in ways that lead them to have more difficulty regulating their emotions and interpreting cues and communication from others. This negatively affects their socialization and may result in a tendency to violence or aggression towards others, among other problem behaviors.[6]

In a national survey conducted in 2008 and 2009, more than 4 in 10 (43%-46%) children (aged 18 months to 17 years) who were placed in a foster family home following an investigation of alleged child abuse and neglect in their families were found at risk of a behavioral or emotional problem and potentially in need of mental health services. Among children of that same age group who were placed in a foster care group home or institution, as many as 7 in 10 (61%-70%) were at such risk.[7] These rates are much higher than those found in the general population. In separate surveys, about 7% to 11% of all children (in roughly the same age range) were identified as having emotional and behavioral problems.[8]

In recent years, children whose Medicaid eligibility is based on their "foster care" status[9] have been increasingly more likely to be given mental health diagnoses.[10] This is also true of children generally.[11] Such diagnoses include attention disorders, anxiety, autism, bipolar disorders, conduct disorders, depression, and schizophrenia.[12] Nearly all children who are in foster care are eligible for health care services funded via Medicaid (as discussed further in the next section).[13] From 2002 to 2007, the share of children whose Medicaid eligibility is based on their "foster care" status who were diagnosed with mental health disorders increased for most of these conditions. The most common diagnoses varied by age and older children were more likely to be given one of these diagnoses. In 2007, children ages 3 to 5 were most likely to have diagnoses of conduct disorder (7.4%) and attention disorders (6.7%); children ages 6 to 11 were most likely to be diagnosed with attention disorders (52.5%) and conduct disorders (26.8%); and children ages 12 to 18 years old were most likely to be diagnosed with conduct disorders (67.3%) and depression (44.4%).[14]

Figure 1 (below) shows, for 2002 and 2007, rates of major mental health diagnoses by age group (6 to 11 years and 12 to 18 years) among children whose Medicaid eligibility is based on their "foster care" status. The figure indicates that these rates went up across all diagnoses for both age groups, except for depression among children ages 6 to 11 and schizophrenia among both age groups.

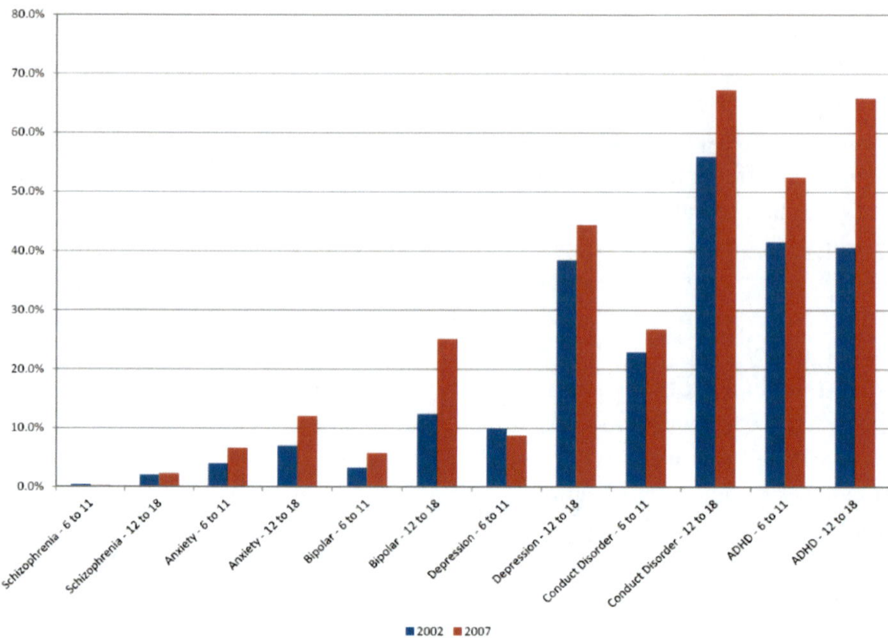

Source: Figure prepared by the Congressional Research Service (CRS) based on data from David Rubin et al., "Interstate Variation in Trends of Psychotropic Medication Use Among Medicaid-enrolled Children in Foster Care," *Child and Youth Services Review*, Vol. 34, No. 8, 2012, p. 1492.

Notes: "ADHD" stands for attention deficit hyperactivity disorder." The report does not define ADHD or other health conditions that were studied. The American Psychiatric Association's Diagnostic and Statistical Manual (DSM) is the standard classification of mental disorders used by mental health professionals, and defines these terms. For further information, see American Psychiatric Association, "DSM," http://www.psychiatry.org/practice/dsm.

Nearly all children in foster care qualify for Medicaid through a designated pathway for this population or through other pathways. The study by Rubin et al., included children as in "foster care" if, in a given year (FY2002 or FY2007), the child had at least one month of Medicaid eligibility under the "foster care child" eligibility pathway. For Medicaid reporting purposes, this includes some (but not all) children in foster care, many children who are adopted from foster care, and certain children who have aged out of foster care. For further information, see CRS Report R42378, *Child Welfare: Health Care Needs of Children in Foster Care and Related Federal Issues*.

Figure 1. Rates of Major Mental Health Diagnoses Among Medicaid-Enrolled Children in Foster Care by Age (6 to 11 years and 12 to 18 years), 2002 and 2007.

Mental Health Services and Treatments for Children in Foster Care

National standards for mental health care developed by leading child welfare and pediatric organizations propose that all children should receive a mental health screening when placed into foster care, a subsequent comprehensive mental health assessment by a mental health professional within a month of being placed into care, and a coordinated approach to delivery of services to meet the children's ongoing mental health needs.[15] Such diagnostic and treatment services should currently be available to children in foster care through Medicaid (Title XIX of the Social Security Act), which is a means-tested entitlement program administered by the federal government in partnership with the states. Under Medicaid, each state designs a plan for provision of medical assistance in its own state, including primary and acute medical services, as well as long-term care. The plan must be consistent with federal requirements and, if approved by HHS, entitles the state to federal reimbursement for a part of the cost of providing that medical assistance to each eligible individual in the state.

Most, if not all, children in foster care are eligible for Medicaid[16] and are generally entitled to the same set of "traditional" Medicaid state plan services available to other children enrolled in a given state's Medicaid program. Central among these benefits is a provision in the law requiring that children receive all medically necessary services authorized in federal statute through the Early and Periodic Screening, Diagnosis, and Treatment (EPSDT) program. The EPSDT program covers health screenings and services, including assessments of each child's physical and mental health development; laboratory tests (including lead blood level assessment); appropriate immunizations; health education; and vision, dental, and hearing services. The screenings and services must be provided at regular intervals that meet "reasonable" medical or dental practice standards. Under EPSDT, states are required to provide treatment to meet children's identified health needs, including mental health needs.[17] Medicaid financing may be used to provide services to meet children's behavioral health needs, including case management or services provided by psychiatrists, psychologists, or clinical social workers. It may also be used to pay for prescription drugs.[18]

In general, children who have mental health challenges may benefit from health care services that could include psychosocial treatment, such as counseling and case management from mental health professionals. There is a growing body of evidence on practices for responding to mental disorders in children through the use of psychosocial treatment. For example, certain psychosocial treatment interventions (i.e., behavioral and cognitive-behavioral therapy [CBT]; family-focused and group-based treatment; and treatments with multiple types of interventions) have been found to be moderately effective for children or parents of children with antisocial-related and disruptive behaviors.[19] In addition, CBT—such as activities that include anger management, conflict resolution, and social skills training—has been found to be effective for children who experience trauma (defined as actual or threatened death or serious injury, or a threat to the physical integrity of self or others).[20]

A medical professional may prescribe psychotropic medications to children in foster care when psychosocial treatment alone is not effective or when pharmaceutical or combination treatment has been demonstrated to be more effective than psychosocial treatment.[21] Nonetheless, psychotropics may still be prescribed without accompanying psychosocial therapies because medical professionals and other stakeholders may not have resources and support readily available to address the complex mental health needs of children in care.[22]

Analysis of data from a national survey of children who come into contact with child welfare agencies due to investigation of alleged child abuse or neglect found that children entering foster care were more likely to receive supports (i.e., mental health screening, a follow-up mental health assessment by a mental health professional, and referral to services) than were children with mental health needs who remained in their own homes following such an investigation. Even so, receipt of these services was not universal among those entering care. About 8 out of 10 children entering care received services consistent with at least one of the three services outlined by the national standards.[23]

Other studies have shown that children in foster care who need mental health services do not always receive them.[24] A national survey that collected data between 2008 and 2010 found that among children who had been in foster care for approximately 18 months or less, and who met clinical criteria for a mental health need, 3 out of 10 did not receive any specialty mental health services (e.g., counseling or residential or outpatient treatments) or psychotropics, and another 9% received psychotropics without any such services.[25] (See Figure 2.)

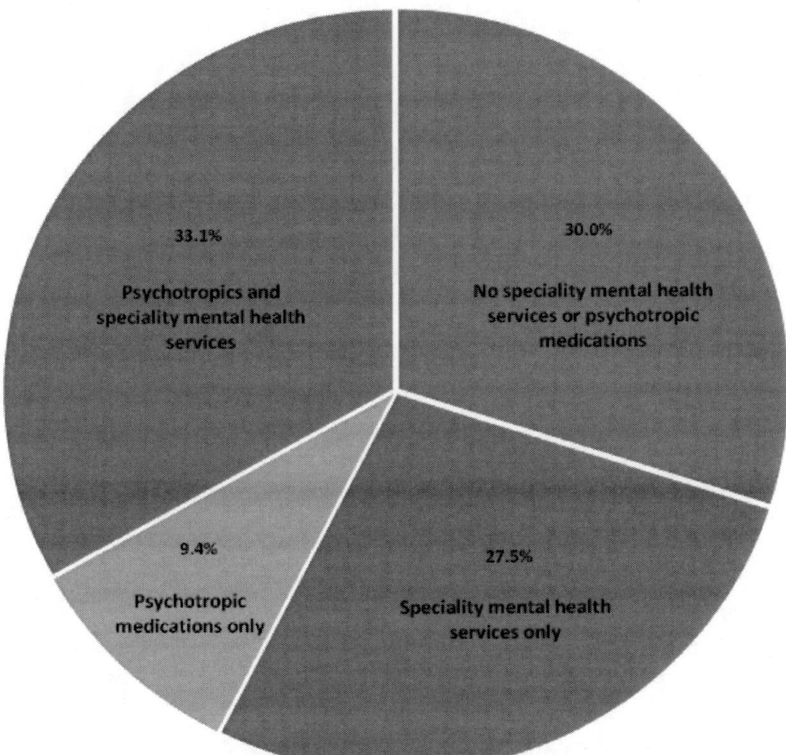

Source: Figure prepared by the Congressional Research Service (CRS) based on data from Leyla F. Stambaugh et al., *Psychotropic Medication Use by Children in Child Welfare*, U.S. Department of Health and Human Services, Administration for Children and Families, Office of Planning, Research, and Evaluation, National Survey of Child and Adolescent Well-Being Report, No. 17, 2012.

Notes: These data are based on a subset of the overall sample of children in the survey who were involved in child welfare. Interviews were conducted with caregivers approximately 18 months after the investigation of child abuse or neglect that brought the child to the attention of the child welfare agency. Foster care refers to a foster family home, a formal kinship placement, and a group home or residential program. In a formal kinship care living arrangement, the caregiver receives some financial support for being a foster parent. A group home or residential program refers to a congregate care setting. Specialty mental health services can include services such as seeing a private mental health professional or family doctor mental health service, in-home counseling or crisis services, mental health or community health centers, outpatient drug or alcohol clinics, or a psychiatric unit in a hospital, among other services.

Figure 2. Share of Children in Foster Care (Ages 16 Months to19 Years Old Who Met Clinical Criteria for a Mental Health Need) and Their Use of Psychotropics and Specialty Mental Health Services; Percentages based on caregiver reports at time of interview or youth self-report for those 18 or older.

USE OF PSYCHOTROPIC DRUGS BY CHILDREN IN FOSTER CARE

Between 16% and 33% of children in out-of-home care may be using psychotropic medication on any given day, although the rate of use varies significantly based on certain factors, including the child's age, placement setting, and length of involvement with the child welfare agency.[26] Rates of psychotropic medication use among children in foster care far exceed the rates among children generally, which is about 6%.[27] Children whose Medicaid eligibility is based on their foster care status have been found to receive psychotropic medication at three to nine times the rate of all other children served by Medicaid,[28] and at a level that is somewhat comparable to (but still higher than) older children (ages 13 to 18) with a diagnosed mental disorder or neurodevelopmental disorder.[29] At the same time, research based on a national study of the use of outpatient mental health services found that children living in non-relative foster family homes were no more likely than those living in their own homes to be prescribed psychotropic medication. (Importantly, this study does not include children in foster care group settings or residential treatment facilities, who tend to have higher rates of psychotropic use.)[30]

Variations by State and Over Time

Rates of psychotropic medication use among children involved with the child welfare system, including those in foster care, vary by state and over time. Research from the early 2000s found great variation in prescription of psychotropic medication for children involved with the child welfare system, including those in foster care. Closer analysis of the differences across states led the researchers to conclude that differences in risk for mental health services was not the primary factor leading to variation, suggesting the importance of state practices in prescribing psychotropic medication.[31]

A separate study of Medicaid claims data from 2002 to 2007 showed variation among psychotropic medication use among children whose eligibility for Medicaid was based on their "foster care" status.[32] The study found an initial increase in the use of psychotropic medications followed by some decline in most states. However, across this same time frame the study found an increase in the use of antipsychotic medications—which are a subset of psychotropic drugs generally used to treat schizophrenia and sometimes bipolar disorder—among children whose Medicaid eligibility was based on their "foster care" status. Specifically, it found that 45 states experienced a relative increase in the use of these medications from 2002 to 2007, two states experienced a relative decrease, and one state experienced no change over the period. In 2007, the annual rate of antipsychotic medication use among children in foster care ranged from 2.8% to 21.7% in each state.[33]

Findings from the Second National Survey of Child and Adolescent Well-Being (NSCAW)

This section uses data primarily from the second National Survey on Child and Adolescent Well-Being (NSCAW II) to provide a more detailed discussion of psychotropic medication use among children in foster care.

NSCAW II examined the outcomes of a national sample of 5,872 children who came into contact with the child welfare system through an investigation of child abuse or neglect in their homes, including the extent to which these children were prescribed psychotropic medications.[34] The survey captured the experiences of children in this sample who remained in their homes following the investigation (including those children who stayed with their biological or adoptive parents and those who lived informally with relatives) and those who were removed from their homes and placed in foster care (including children who were placed in a non-relative foster family home, those placed formally with kin, and those who went to live in a group home or a residential program). At the time of the initial NSCAW II Survey, 4 to 6 months after the initial investigation (in 2008-2009), these children's ages ranged from 2 months to 17.5 years. At the time of the 18- month follow-up (in 2009-2011), they were 16 months to 19 years; and at the 36-month follow-up (2011-2012), they were ages 34 months to 20 years old.[35] Children in the sample were not necessarily in foster care for the entire 18- or 36-month period. They may have entered and reentered care, or they could have entered care after a subsequent investigation.

As discussed in the following sections, the NSCAW II data show that children living with their own parents following an investigation of child abuse or neglect were less likely to be using psychotropic medication than those living in foster care at that time. Among children who were in foster care, living in a congregate care and being school age forecast a greater chance that a child in foster care was taking psychotropic medications.[36]

Living at Home vs. Living out of Home

Among children in the NSCAW II study, there was not a statistically significant difference in the use of psychotropic medications among those who, at four to six months following the investigation, were placed in foster care (15.9%) and those who had remained in their homes (11.6%). However, at 18 months following the investigation, children in foster care were significantly more likely to be taking psychotropic medications than those who remained in their homes (23.1% vs. 10.9%). At the 36-month follow-up, more than one out of three children in care (32.8%) was taking psychotropics, compared to 12.9% of children who remained in their homes. (For more information, see Appendix A.)[37]

Placement Setting

Among children placed in foster care, psychotropic medication use was significantly greater for those who lived in foster group homes or residential treatment programs than among those in foster family homes and formal kin care. Prevalence among children in group foster care settings was close to one-half (48.2%) for children who had been in care for six months or less after the initial investigation of child abuse or neglect. This is compared to 11.8% to 19.5% of children in the foster care settings.[38]

Figure 3 shows the rate of psychotropic medication use by whether children lived out of home, or for children in foster care, all placement settings approximately 18 months after the initial investigation of child abuse or neglect.[39] As with the earlier wave (six months or less after the investigation), those in group settings were most likely to be prescribed psychotropics (67.4%), compared to less than a quarter of children in other foster care settings (15.9% to 23.8%), children who remained in their own homes (10.9%), and informal kin care (11.9%). This pattern held true 36 months after the investigation for child abuse and neglect (not shown in the figure). Just over half of children in group settings were taking psychotropics (52%). The rate of use was 16.5% to 36.1% among children in other types of foster care settings; 12.5% for children who remained in their own homes; and 16.5% for those who were in informal kin care.[40]

Concurrent Use of Psychotropic Medications

Figure 3 also displays the frequency with which children involved in the child welfare system were taking more than one psychotropic medication, by placement setting, approximately 18 months after the initial investigation. Compared to children in other placement settings, children in foster care group homes or residential settings were most likely to be taking more than one psychotropic medication. About half of foster children in group settings (48.6%) who were prescribed psychotropics were taking two or more drugs, whereas the rate of children in other child welfare settings taking two or more drugs was 5.7% to 14.6%.[41]

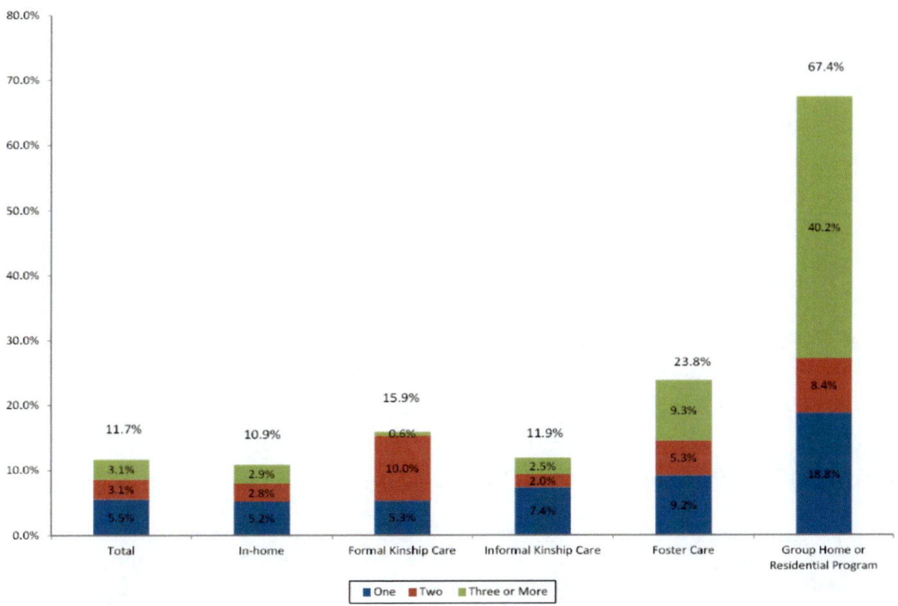

Source: Figure prepared by the Congressional Research Service (CRS) based on data from Cecilia Casanueva et al., *NSCAW II Wave 2 Report: Children's Services,* Exhibit 14, Final Report, RTI International for U.S. Department of Health and Human Services, Administration for Children and Families, Office of Planning, Research and Evaluation, July 2012.

Notes: Interviews were conducted with caregivers approximately 18 months after the investigation of child abuse or neglect that brought the child to the attention of the child welfare agency. In-home refers to children who were not removed from the home of their parents following an investigation for abuse and neglect. Kinship care refers to living with a relative caregiver, such as a grandparent, aunt, uncle, or other relative. In a formal kinship care living arrangement, the relative caregiver receives some financial support for being a foster parent. Foster care refers to a nonrelative foster family home, and group home or residential program refers to a congregate care setting.

Figure 3. Current Use of Psychotropic Medication by All Children Who Come Into Contact with Child Welfare Services, by Placement Type, and Number of Psychotropic Medications; Percentage based on caregivers report at time of interview.

At 36 months following the initial investigation (not shown in the figure), about 4 of 10 children in group settings were taking two or more psychotropic medications, followed by children in foster care (18.2%), formal kin care (11.1%), informal kin care (8.8%), and those who remained in their own homes (7.2%). Children in group settings were significantly more likely to be using three or more psychotropic medications at 36 months following the investigation than children in all other settings.[42]

Age of Children in Foster Care

In general, children in foster care were more likely to be using psychotropic medication if they were of elementary and secondary school age. Figure 4 shows that at each wave (4 to 6 months after investigation, 18 month follow-up, and 36 month follow-up), youth ages 11 to 17 were most likely to be using psychotropics. This is followed by youth ages 6 to 10, youth ages 18 and older, and youth ages 1.5 to 5 years. Notably, the oldest youth, those ages 18 and older, were not as likely to be taking psychotropic medications as children ages 6 through 17.

Prescribing Patterns: "Too Many, Too Much, and Too Young"

The research literature has characterized patterns of prescribing psychotropic drugs to foster children as "too many, too much, and too young."[43] "Too many" refers to children taking multiple psychotropic medications at a time. An analysis of national Medicaid claims data from 2002 through 2007 found that polypharmacy—defined in the analysis as concurrent use of three or more psychotropic medication classes for at least 30 days during a one-year period—was fairly consistent over that period, at about 5.2% to 5.9%, annually, among all children whose eligibility for Medicaid was based on their "foster care" status.[44] Data from the NSCAW II study indicate that for children in foster care who were prescribed psychotropics, the average number of psychotropics per child was 1.9 on a given day.[45]

As discussed previously, Figure 3 illustrates the percentage of children who were prescribed one, two, or three or more psychotropic medications. The difference between the shares of children in group or residential settings who are prescribed three or more psychotropics is statistically significant when compared to the other groups of children. Concerns have been raised about using certain classes of psychotropics, such as antipsychotics, concurrently. Antipsychotic polypharmacy (i.e., use of multiple antipsychotic medications) has not been well researched and has typically demonstrated "greater adverse effects with only marginal benefits."[46]

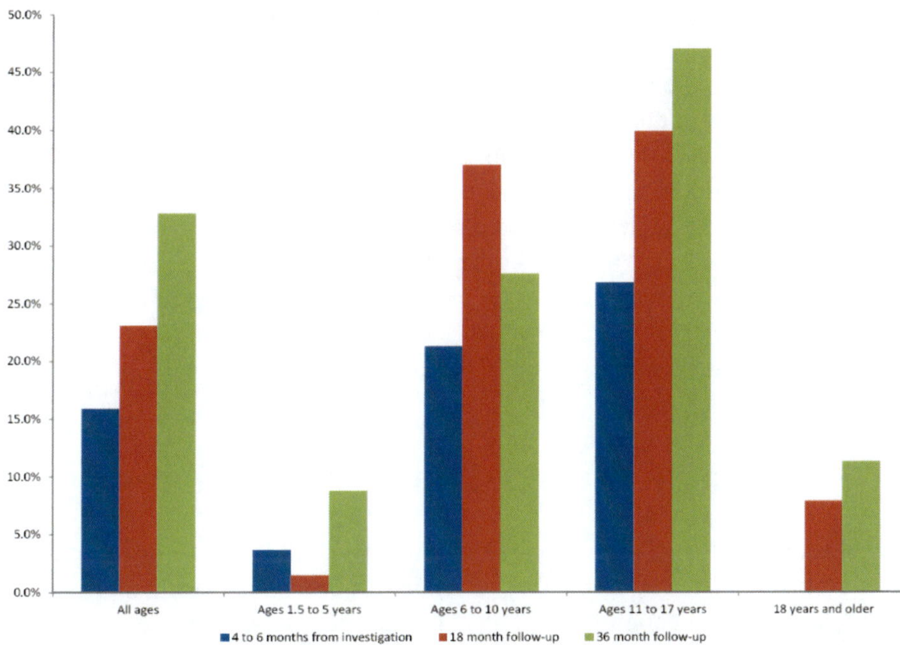

Source: Figure prepared by the Congressional Research Service (CRS) based on data from Cecilia Casanueva et al., *NSCAW II Wave 2 Report: Children's Services,* Exhibit 14, Final Report, RTI International for U.S. Department of Health and Human Services, Administration for Children and Families, Office of Planning, Research and Evaluation, July 2012.

Notes: Children in the sample were not necessarily in foster care for the entire 18- or 36-month period. They may have entered and re-entered care during this time, or they could have entered care after a subsequent investigation. In-home refers to children who were not removed from the home of their parents following an investigation for abuse and neglect. Kinship care refers to living with a relative caregiver, such as a grandparent, aunt, uncle, or other relative. In a formal kinship care living arrangement, the relative caregiver receives some financial support for being a foster parent. Foster care refers to a nonrelative foster family home, and group home or residential program refers to a congregate care setting.

Figure 4. Current Use of Psychotropic Medication by All Children Who Come Into Contact with Child Welfare Services, by Age and Time From Initial Investigation; Percentage based on caregiver report at time of interview or youth self-report for those age 18 or older.

Further, "too much" refers to the prescriptions for foster children in dosages that exceed recommendations. This is of particular concern because, as discussed above, studies on the safety and efficacy of these medications for children are limited. Finally, "too young" refers to concerns that very young children are prescribed psychotropics. The NSCAW II study found that 2.2% of children under the age of 6 in out-of-home care (foster care, formal kinship care, or group home and residential programs) were prescribed psychotropics.[47] A 2011 GAO report examined the use of psychotropic drugs among foster children in five states, and found that in each of these states 0.3% to 2.1% of children under age 1 were prescribed psychotropics, compared to a lower rate (0.1% to 1.2%) of infants of the same age who were not in foster care. Health experts have raised concerns that there are no established mental health indications for the use of psychotropic drugs in infants, and that psychotropics use by infants can lead to serious health effects.[48]

WEIGHING THE BENEFITS OF PSYCHOTROPICS

Because children in foster care tend to have greater mental health service needs than other children, they may be more likely to benefit from psychotropic medications. Still, as mentioned previously, psychotropic medications may not be effective in treating the mental health needs of some individuals.

Children in care may more readily receive psychotropics due to the paucity of psychosocial services available. This could be due to a number of factors, including a shortage of mental health providers generally and of those who have clinical understanding of the complex trauma many children in foster care may have experienced and/or who specialize in therapies that have proven to be effective.[49] While the rate of prescribing psychotropics has decreased in recent years, the use of certain classes of these drugs—namely antipsychotics, used for the off-label treatment[50] of children who have bipolar disorders and schizophrenia, and used to treat certain other behavioral conditions—has steadily grown. As discussed previously, the share of children in foster care prescribed antipsychotic medication increased from 2002 to 2007, with an average change across states of 12.8% over this period. This increase could be due to a number of factors, including more research (albeit limited) on the efficacy of these medications in children and the role of pharmaceutical companies marketing drugs to prescribers and consumers.[51]

Further, children generally have increasingly been prescribed certain psychotropic medications in recent years.[52]

The use of psychotropics by children in foster care has come under growing scrutiny by policymakers and stakeholders in the child welfare field. Although there is an expanding body of research on psychotropic use among children with mental health disorders, few studies show that they are safe and effective for this population. A review by the Department of Health and Human Services (HHS) of research on one class of psychotropics, antipsychotics, found that most studies had insufficient evidence to draw a conclusion about the safety of these drugs in addressing child mental health disorders generally—*not just those occurring among foster youth*. Further, little to no evidence was available for certain conditions such as disruptive behavior disorders, obsessive compulsive disorders, or eating disorders (i.e., anorexia nervosa). According to the analysis, the median study duration of eight weeks was insufficient to evaluate some long-term outcomes. The analysis also found that most of the studies had a high risk of bias because missing data were not handled and reported properly, study participants were not randomly assigned to the treatment groups, and/or the studies were funded by pharmaceutical companies that manufacture the psychotropic medication.[53] Other research has shown that antipsychotics are associated with harmful health outcomes in some children, including high cholesterol levels, weight gain, and type-2 diabetes.[54]

Despite these concerns, some children in foster care may benefit from psychotropic medication for managing symptoms and issues associated with mental health and behavior concerns stemming from their exposure to complex trauma, particularly if this treatment is coupled with psychosocial services.[55] Stimulants for the treatment of attention deficit hyperactivity disorder (ADHD), a common childhood disorder, appear to be among the best researched of the antipsychotic classes. Multiple studies with research methodologies that used randomized control trials have found that some stimulants are very effective at reducing the core symptoms of ADHD, including hyperactivity, impulsivity, inattention, and aggression.[56]

Further, children in foster care are more likely to have a mental health diagnosis than children generally, including children who are low income. A 2011 Government Accountability Office (GAO) report on psychotropic medication use by children in foster care cited statements from state officials and child psychiatrists that higher levels of psychotropic drug use may be appropriate to deal with the increased prevalence and greater severity of mental health conditions among this population. In addition, multiple foster care placements and inconsistent state oversight practices for managing their care may contribute to the likelihood that psychotropics are used to respond to the mental health needs of these children.[57]

CONGRESSIONAL OVERSIGHT

Congress has taken a strong interest in oversight of prescription medications used by children in foster care. In 2005, the House Ways and Means Subcommittee on Human Resources held a hearing to examine the enrollment of children in foster care in clinical drug trials. The hearing followed media reports concerning use of foster children in clinical AIDS drug trials and addressed the extent to which states properly oversee prescription drug use by children in foster care.[58] As part of the Child and Family Services Improvement Act of 2006 (P.L. 109-288), Congress required state child welfare agencies, as a condition of receiving certain child welfare funding, to describe how they actively consulted with physicians or other medical professionals in assessing the health and well-being of children in foster care and in determining appropriate medical treatment for them.[59]

The issue of oversight of psychotropic medication use for children in foster care in particular was briefly discussed at a 2007 congressional hearing on health care oversight for children in foster care, and it was the sole topic of a 2008 hearing (both held by the Ways and Means Subcommittee on Income Security and Family Support[60]).[61] Subsequently, as part of the Fostering Connections to Success and Increasing Adoptions Act of 2008 (P.L. 110-351), Congress expanded on the requirement that states consult with medical professionals on the health and well-being of children in foster care. Specifically, states are required through their child welfare and Medicaid agencies, and in consultation with appropriate medical professionals, to develop a coordinated strategy and oversight plan to ensure access to health care, including mental health services for each child in foster care. The 2008 law directed states to ensure this coordinated strategy provided for oversight of drugs prescribed to children in foster care. In October 2011, the Child and Family Services Improvement and Innovation Act (P.L. 112-34) amended this provision to further stipulate that the coordinated strategy must include protocols for use of psychotropic medication for children in foster care.

In December 2011, the Senate Homeland Security and Governmental Affairs Subcommittee on Federal Financial Management, Government Information, Federal Services and International Security held an oversight hearing[62] that focused on the results and recommendations of the aforementioned study by the Government Accountability Office. GAO reviewed state policies and regulations for oversight of prescribing psychotropic medications in six states.[63] The study compared state policies against best practice guidelines for prescribing psychotropics for foster children and other vulnerable child populations. These best practice guidelines were developed by the American Academy of Child and Adolescent Psychiatry (AACAP) in consultation with the Substance Abuse and Mental Health Services Administration (SAMHSA) at HHS.[64] Overall, GAO found that each of the six state programs falls short of providing comprehensive oversight as defined by AACAP. For example, though all six states implemented some practices consistent with the guidelines for consent procedures, only one state (Texas) fully implemented these procedures.[65] According to the report, states that do not incorporate consent procedures similar to AACAP's guidelines may increase the likelihood that caregivers are not fully aware of the risks and benefits associated with the decision to use psychotropic medications.

Witnesses at the hearing spoke about the role of HHS and the state Medicaid programs in increasing cooperation and communication between the agencies and discussed how HHS could increase the guidance on best practices to assist states in preparing plans for psychotropic medication oversight. Further, a 12-year-old former foster youth described being given multiple mental health diagnoses and side effects he experienced from multiple psychotropic medications that were prescribed to him while in foster care. He also testified that a therapist that he saw with his adoptive parents was most helpful to him.

Additionally, in April 2013 the Senate Finance Committee convened a roundtable discussion with Senate staff and child welfare stakeholders to address issues associated with the prescription of psychotropic medications for children in foster care and to highlight alternative strategies to effectively respond to trauma experienced by children and youth in foster care. At the roundtable, current and former foster youth shared their experiences with psychotropic medication and some noted that therapy ultimately helped them transition from psychotropic medications. The youths' stories sometimes highlighted the importance of an invested caregiver or other knowledgeable professional in ensuring that appropriate mental health treatment is identified and provided. Child welfare stakeholders discussed the prevalence of psychotropic medication use among subpopulations of youth; the role of the federal government in promoting alternatives to psychotropics; tools for determining whether youth should be prescribed medications; and the roles of schools, the mental health system, and foster parents in engaging with youth on whether psychotropic medications should be prescribed.

Finally, in May 2014 the House Ways and Means Subcommittee on Human Resources held a hearing on the use of psychotropic medications among children in foster care and the efforts of states and the federal government to ensure that such medications are used appropriately. Witnesses included the Associate Commissioner of HHS's Children's Bureau; GAO; a researcher who focuses on psychotropic medication use among children in care; and Dr. Phil McGraw, who has sought to bring greater awareness to the issue.[66]

RECENT EXECUTIVE BRANCH ACTIONS

The Administration has proposed expanding funding for oversight of psychotropic medications as part of the FY2016 budget, which, as of the date of this report, has not been enacted. In addition, several federal agencies have worked both together and independently to help gain a better understanding of psychotropic medication use among children (especially children in foster care). As part of their efforts to promote interagency cooperation, they have publicized best practices and successful state strategies related to the oversight of psychotropic medication use for children and the development of alternative strategies for children with mental health needs.

FY2016 Request: Demonstration to Address "Over-Prescription" of Psychotropic Medication for Children in Foster Care[67]

The President's budget proposes a five-year joint initiative between CMS and ACF to reduce reliance on psychotropic medications for children in foster care and improve their well-being. This would be accomplished by providing performance-based incentive payments to state Medicaid agencies (total of $500 million in incentive funding across five years, FY2016-FY2020) that meet certain outcomes or other requirements related to improved care coordination and delivery of evidence-based psychosocial interventions to Medicaid-eligible children who are also served by child welfare agencies.

Incentive payments would be paid annually out of the Medicaid program (Title XIX of the Social Security Act) over the five-year periodm.[68]

States could also apply, through the state child welfare agency, for competitive grant funding under the Title IV-E Foster Care program (total of $250 million across five years, FY2016- FY2020) to build state capacity and infrastructure to implement alternative psychosocial interventions. ACF funding would support activities that include child welfare funding for training of caregivers and caseworkers on mental health needs of children in care, screening and assessment tools, coordination between the child welfare and Medicaid systems, and fidelity monitoring of implementation of evidence-based intervention.[69]

Federal Interagency Working Group Established

In the summer of 2011, HHS convened an interagency working group to address emerging research on the use of psychotropic medication among children in foster care and to support state efforts in implementing the requirements on psychotropics in P.L. 112-34. The working group is led by the Administration for Children and Families (ACF), which administers child welfare programs, and includes representatives from other HHS agencies, including the Centers for Medicare and Medicaid Services (CMS) and the Substance Abuse and Mental Health Services Administration (SAMHSA). The working group developed a plan to expand the use of evidence-based screening, diagnosis, and interventions; strengthen the oversight and monitoring of psychotropic medications; and expand the research evidence regarding medications and psychosocial treatments for children in foster care.[70]

State Interagency Cooperation and Collaboration Promoted

In November 2011, three agencies in the working group—ACF, SAMHSA, and CMS—released a letter addressed to the directors of each state child welfare, Medicaid, and mental health agency. The letter addressed actions being taken at the three federal agencies to "support effective management" of prescription medication use for children in foster care.[71] According to the letter, "State Medicaid/CHIP agencies and mental health authorities play a significant role in providing continuous access to and receipt of quality mental health services for children in out-of-home care. Therefore it is essential that State child welfare, Medicaid, and mental health authorities collaborate in any efforts to improve health, including medication use and prescription monitoring structures in particular." The letter further discussed other steps the agencies would take to raise awareness about psychotropic use among children in foster care.

ACF, SAMHSA, and CMS (in partnership with their training and technical assistance providers) subsequently took steps to provide guidance to states and other stakeholders on oversight of psychotropics through a series of webinars and information memoranda. In January and February 2012, they held webinars for child welfare and other stakeholders that presented data, research, and practices for monitoring and oversight of psychotropic medication use among children in foster care.[72] In addition, the three agencies held a series of question and answer discussion sessions in March through June 2012 for state child welfare and mental health leaders who are working together on plans to enhance oversight and monitoring.[73]

In late August 2012, HHS (ACF, SAMHSA, and CMS) convened state directors of child welfare, Medicaid, and mental health agencies to address the use of psychotropic medications for children in foster care and the mental health needs of children who have experienced trauma. The summit, "Because Minds Matter," was intended to provide an opportunity for state leaders to enhance their collaboration on the appropriate use of psychotropic medications.[74] They were asked to examine what aspects of oversight needed improvement and the steps needed to implement changes. States were also asked to outline the activities they would undertake to meet their goals, the anticipated challenges, the necessary partners, and a timeline for implementation.[75] The summit included multiple presentations from HHS staff, researchers, and selected state teams about a range of psychotropic oversight and related topics.[76]

Since the summit, HHS has furthered its work in this area. For example, ACF awarded FY2012 funds to nine entities (state and county child welfare agencies, universities, and a children's hospital) to support projects intended to provide assistance to youth in child welfare who have mental and behavioral health needs using evidence-based intervention models.[77] ACF also awarded FY2013 funds to six entities (state child welfare agencies, universities, and a children's organization) to promote well-being after children experience trauma.[78]

Professional Protocols and Other State Best Practices Disseminated

In April 2012, ACF provided guidance to state child welfare agencies on implementing protocols to monitor the use of psychotropic medication. As part of this guidance, HHS synthesized information about use of psychotropics based on guidelines issued by child welfare and medical professionals.[79] These elements address coordinated planning, informed and shared decision-making, medication monitoring, mental health expertise and consultation, and mechanisms for sharing accurate and up-to-date information.[80] (As discussed in a subsequent section, HHS requires that states report on the extent to which these elements are in place as part of their monitoring of psychotropic drug use for children in foster care.) ACF also issued separate guidance in April 2012 to state child welfare agencies about the ways they can focus on improving the behavioral and social-emotional outcomes for children who have experienced abuse and/or neglect. The guidance discussed the emerging evidence on the impact of maltreatment in terms of its effect on brain development as it affects a child's social and emotional development. It also outlined the federal child welfare and Medicaid requirements (including those discussed in this report) around meeting the emotional and behavioral needs of children in foster care, and the ways in which states and child welfare agencies can respond to these needs.[81]

The CMS Center for Medicaid and CHIP Services issued an informational bulletin in August 2012 to make states aware of resources and opportunities to address the use of psychotropic medication in vulnerable populations, including children in foster care. The informational bulletin noted that all states are required to have Drug Utilization Review programs in place to oversee the prescribing of drugs for Medicaid beneficiaries and provided examples of the way some states have used this review to provide oversight of psychotropic medication use. For example, automated system "edit checks" may be used to ensure prescriptions are consistent with accepted medical practice (e.g., special authorization must be granted for prescriptions of children younger than a given age). The bulletin alternatively noted that some states have multidisciplinary teams (drawing from public and private entities) to review cases and ensure appropriate prescription of psychotropics. Further, the bulletin advised states that "robust screening and assessment practices that are attentive to trauma and social/emotional functions, careful and coordinated treatment planning, and the judicious and thoughtful use of all treatment options available to the youth, especially those with a strong evidence base" are practices most likely to support health and wellbeing of youth in foster care who have potential behavioral health problems.[82]

CMS, ACF, and SAMHSA issued joint guidance in July 2013 to convey the importance of making psychosocial interventions available to children who have experienced "complex trauma"—described in the guidance as "children's exposure to multiple or prolonged traumatic events, which are often invasive and interpersonal in nature"—and to highlight how states may use existing federal funding and authority to provide those interventions. The guidance noted that children in foster care may be more likely to receive psychotropic medication, and may not be prescribed psychotropics properly, because of the complexity of their symptoms and the lack of appropriate screening, assessment, and treatment. The guidance promoted the use of functional assessments (periodic evaluation of a child's well-being using standardized, valid, and reliable measurement tools), trauma screening (brief evaluation of potential trauma symptoms and/or history), mental health assessment (in-depth clinical evaluation of an individual's mental health status), and outcome measurement and progress monitoring (measuring success by tracking child-level well-being outcomes to ensure treatment services are achieving desired improvements in children's health and functioning).

Finally, the July 2013 interagency guidance discusses existing federal programs and policies in each of three systems (child welfare, mental health, and Medicaid) that can be used to serve children with mental health treatment needs associated with complex trauma. These include funding for services provided to state child welfare agencies under Title IV-B (of the Social Security Act), which among many other things may be used to fund family or individual counseling that responds to the trauma-related needs of children involved in child welfare. Further, child welfare agencies can use Title IV-E funding under the Social Security Act to support child welfare training concerning the nature and consequences of child trauma, the use of screening and assessment tools, and evidence-based practices to address trauma. (However, Title IV-E training dollars may not be used to train workers to provide services that respond to children's mental health needs.) Medicaid offers states a way to finance screenings, assessments, behavioral health services, therapy, and case management for children with complex trauma needs (many of these services are mandatory for eligible children), and it may also be used to pay for prescription drugs. Finally, SAMHSA administers block grant funding that may support non-Medicaid covered treatment services, and it supports other technical assistance and projects related to understanding trauma experienced by children and providing evidence-based and effective treatment.[83]

STATE OVERSIGHT EFFORTS

Recent studies have focused on the role of states in overseeing the use of psychotropic medication for children in foster care. For example, some research has addressed the issue of obtaining consent for using psychotropics or examining how certain states are carrying out their monitoring procedures.[84] Researchers have also conducted surveys of states to learn about their policies related to the oversight of psychotropic medications. Some of these surveys predate the specific requirement for oversight of prescription medications and others have been conducted since then; however, none of these surveys address how states have responded to the federal provision (added to the law in September 2011) on oversight of psychotropic medications specifically.

In 2009 and 2010, researchers surveyed states to learn about the status of policies and guidelines for overseeing the use of psychotropic medication by children in foster care, as well as related challenges and solutions that were identified by states. Researchers collected information from 48 states, including the District of Columbia. Of the states surveyed, more than half (58.7%) rated psychotropic medication use to be of high concern (a rating of 8 to 10 on a scale of 1 to 10). About a quarter of the states rated the issue of moderate concern (a rating of 5 to 7), and about 13% rated it of low concern (a rating of 1 to 4). At the time of the survey, 26 of the 48 states had a written policy or guideline regarding psychotropic medication use; 13 states were currently developing a policy or guideline; and 9 states had no policy or guideline. Slightly more than half of states used at least a "red flag" marker to identify problems with the safety and quality of psychotropic drug use. Red flags that states described using included the use of psychotropic medications in young children, the use of multiple medications before the use of a single medication, use of multiple psychotropic medications simultaneously, use of multiple medications within the same class for longer than 30 days, and dosage exceeding current maximum recommendations. Researchers concluded that states were implementing a wide variety of approaches, and that there was little evidence that these approaches were being implemented or studied in a systematic way to identify which approaches helped improve outcomes for children in foster care.[85]

On the other hand, researchers have raised concerns about the availability of policies and procedures that respond to psychotropic medication use. As reported in a 2014 study, these researchers reviewed the statutes, rules, and statements of policies on oversight of psychotropic drug use among children in care from 16 states (which have 72% of all children in care nationally). They were unable to locate many of the policies that had been reported in other studies, and when they did exist, the policies were "extremely underdeveloped and failed to include many of the 'red flag' criteria that both experts and states identified as essential to protecting children, such as the use of psychotropic medication for young children, dosage level, and whether multiple psychotropic medications were prescribed simultaneously."[86]

CURRENT FEDERAL REQUIREMENTS RELATED TO THE OVERSIGHT OF HEALTH CARE FOR CHILDREN IN FOSTER CARE

As noted above, under the Stephanie Tubbs Jones Child Welfare Services Program (Title IV-B, Subpart 1 of the Social Security Act) states must develop a coordinated strategy and oversight plan to ensure access to health care, including mental health services and dental care, for all children in foster care. This coordinated strategy and oversight plan must be developed via a collaborative effort between the state child welfare agency and the state agency that administers Medicaid, in consultation with pediatric and other health care experts, as well as experts in, or recipients of, child welfare services.[87] The coordinated strategy must outline

- a schedule for initial and follow-up health screenings that meet reasonable standards of medical practice;
- how health needs identified through screenings, including emotional trauma associated with a child's maltreatment and removal from home, will be monitored and treated;
- how medical information for children in care will be updated and appropriately shared, which may include the development and implementation of an electronic health record;
- steps to ensure continuity of health care services, which may include the establishment of a medical home for every child in care;

- *the oversight of prescription medicines, including protocols for the appropriate use and monitoring of psychotropic medications* (italics added for emphasis);
- how the state actively consults with and involves physicians or other appropriate medical or nonmedical professionals in assessing the health and well-being of children in foster care and in determining appropriate medical treatment for the children; and
- steps to ensure that the components of the transition plan development process related to the health care needs of children aging out of foster care are met.

Additionally, federal child welfare law requires that the state child welfare agency have a written plan for each child in foster care, including certain health-related records. These records must include the names and addresses of the child's health providers, a record of the child's immunizations, information about the child's medication, and any other relevant health information concerning the child.[88] These records must be reviewed, updated, and supplied to a child's foster care parent or provider at the time of each foster care placement. Additionally, a copy of the record must be provided to a youth at the time he/she leaves care due to age.[89]

STATE PROTOCOLS RELATED TO USE OF PSYCHOTROPIC MEDICATIONS FOR CHILDREN IN FOSTER CARE

The Congressional Research Service (CRS) reviewed state policies on oversight of psychotropic medications. The review looked at the first set of annual reports (known as Annual Progress and Services Reports, or APSRs) submitted by states to HHS following the 2011 enactment of the requirement for protocols specific to psychotropic medication and as such provide a baseline scan of state policy just after the law was changed. The reports are required each year for states seeking federal funds under a number of child welfare programs, including the Stephanie Tubbs Jones Child Welfare Services Program.[90] The 2012 reports that were reviewed by CRS discussed state plans for FY2013 and were the first reports in which HHS required states, consistent with the new requirements added by the Child and Family Services Improvement Act, to describe specific protocols for the appropriate use and monitoring of psychotropic medications for children in foster care (and to identify, through health screenings, whether children have experienced emotional trauma). As shown in the text box below, state oversight protocols must address screening and evaluation to identify mental health needs; consent and assent to treatment and ongoing communication; medication monitoring; availability of mental health expertise; and mechanisms for sharing current information and education materials.[91]

Program Instructions for the Annual Progress and Services Report, 2012

States must submit information to HHS on their plans to provide child and family services by June 30 of each year. The report to be submitted for June 2012 (describing plans for FY2013) was the first in which states were required to provide their protocols for oversight of psychotropic medication use among children in foster care. According to HHS, these protocols were developed from guidelines put forth by the American Academy of Child and Adolescent Psychiatry and the Reach Institute, among others. They include the following:

- Comprehensive and coordinated screening, assessment, and treatment planning mechanisms to identify children's mental health and trauma-treatment needs (including a psychiatric evaluation, as necessary, to identify needs for psychotropic medication).
- Informed and shared decision-making (consent and assent) and methods for ongoing communication between the prescriber, the child, his/her caregivers, other healthcare providers, the child welfare worker, and other key stakeholders.
- Effective medication monitoring at both the client and agency level.
- Availability of mental health expertise and consultation regarding both consent and monitoring issues by a board-certified or board-eligible Child and Adolescent Psychiatrist (at both the agency and individual case level).
- Mechanisms for accessing and sharing accurate and up-to-date information and educational materials related to mental health and trauma-related interventions (including information about psychotropics) to clinicians, child welfare staff, and consumers.

Source: Title IV-B Child and Family Services Plan; Child Abuse Prevention and Treatment State Plan; Chafee Foster Care Independence Program; Educational Training Vouchers Program, ACYF-CB-PI-12-05, April 11, 2012.

CRS Review of State Plans: Process and Limitations

HHS provided CRS with the 2012 APSRs between March and September 2013. The 2012 APSR includes information about state procedures that were in place at least through the submission deadline of June 2012.[92] The review examined portions of the APSR that addressed the five oversight areas shown in the text box above. In addition, CRS used specific search terms, such as "psychotropics" or "medications," to identify other possibly relevant sections of the report. CRS sought to identify common themes within each of the protocols and discuss these across states. If states provided information CRS deemed relevant to more than one protocol, it included this information in its discussion of all relevant protocols. Additionally, in some cases states referenced other state policy manuals or guidance when explaining a protocol for a specific oversight area. CRS reviewed this additional information only when states provided a website address for the document.

CRS's ability to make comparisons across states was limited in a number of ways, including variability in detail, format and style, and reporting by states. In addition, states did not use uniform definitions for some key terms. (For more information about these limitations, see Appendix B.) Additionally, while states may have strengthened their oversight protocols since they submitted the 2012 APSR, this CRS review provides a baseline or benchmark of state procedures immediately after the law changed to require states to have such protocols.

Overview of Findings

Mental Health Screening and Treatment Planning

Thirty states indicated that they provide a mental health evaluation (a screening and/or assessment) for children in care. Ten of these states indicated that they had a trauma screening tool to screen children for traumatic events. The evaluations appear to be available for all children, though some states limit them to children of a minimum age (e.g., age three or older).

States most frequently indicated that evaluations are conducted by the child's primary care physician or a "qualified" (not defined) physician; mental health professional such as a psychiatrist; or staff at community mental health centers, among other types of professionals. States that indicated a time frame for evaluations generally reported that they occur within 30 days of a child being removed from home. Less than half of the states provided information about the steps they take in responding to health care evaluations, which include referrals for services, providing services, and medication.

Consent, Assent, and Ongoing Communication

Thirty-four states provided information concerning their policies related to consent and assent to treatment with psychotropic medication and their methods for ongoing communication between stakeholders involved in the child's health care. States indicated that consent involves one or more of the following parties: a parent/legal guardian, the child, the child welfare agency, and a court/judge. Over half of these states reported that a parent or legal guardian is involved in providing consent. Some states reported requiring a pre-authorization process for the use of psychotropics, in addition to consent or as part of consent. This generally requires the prescriber to submit a request with details about the child, the diagnosis, and the medication to a board, committee, team, or other designated authority that must approve the request before treatment can begin.

Fourteen states provided a description of the information shared among stakeholders as part of the consent process, including type of diagnosis, medication and dosage, benefits or expected results, and potential side effects, among other topics. Most states indicated that a "provider" or "prescriber" could prescribe psychotropic medications. A small number of states were more specific about who could prescribe, indicating that a licensed or licensed and certified physician or a board certified or board eligible specialist in psychiatry, among others, could prescribe psychotropics for children in foster care.

Almost half of all states provided some information about methods for ongoing communication after a child has begun treatment with psychotropic medication. Among others, these include specific databases, a child's medical passport or medical record, and caseworker visits with a child and his/her caregiver family. The types of information shared as a part of ongoing communication include medication details, treatment notes, medical histories, medication benefits or side effects, and changes in medication.

Medication Monitoring

States were asked to describe any written policies related to effective medication monitoring at both the client and agency level. Thirty-six states provided information about monitoring use of psychotropic medication at the client level. States described monitoring both the child and the child's prescriptions.

Monitoring of the child is primarily focused on determining how the medication is affecting him/her. States most frequently mentioned monitoring for side effects and whether targeted symptoms have improved, remained the same, or deteriorated. Thirty-six states described processes used to monitor how medication is affecting an individual child, such as through conversations between the child and caregiver and between the child, caregiver, and caseworker; and logs maintained by the caregiver.

Twenty-five states provided information about medication monitoring at the agency level. Such monitoring can be conducted by the child welfare agency, the overall health program for children in foster care, or special committees or review boards. These entities examined specific aspects of prescribing patterns or trends that they track such as rates of polypharmacy,[93] types of medications, or the number of children receiving medications.

Availability of "Board-Certified" Child and Adolescent Psychiatrists

States did not provide a great deal of detail about the availability of mental health expertise and consultation. Most of the information provided addresses the availability of mental health expertise for individual children rather than for the child welfare agency overall. Seven states specifically reported having access to "board-certified" or "board-eligible" child and adolescent psychiatrists for consultation or review related to the use of psychotropic medication. Thirteen states reported having access to a psychiatrist, a child/adolescent psychiatrist, or a psychiatric consultation service but did not specifically use the term "board-certified" or "board-eligible." Several states generally described the role of the psychiatrist or psychiatric consultation service for an individual child, as well as the specific ways that psychiatrists are involved in consent and monitoring for individual children. Three states described how psychiatrists provide consultation at the agency level.

Education and Training about Psychotropics

Finally, 35 states provided some information about mechanisms for accessing and sharing accurate and up-to-date information and educational materials. These included training, publications, or other materials about psychotropic medications. The 35 states indicated that training is available for child welfare staff; clinicians; and other child welfare stakeholders, including foster parents, staff at residential facilities, juvenile justice agency staff, and children's advocacy groups. States generally did not indicate that information and educational materials are provided to children in care, although one state indicated that it had plans to provide information to foster children.

More detailed findings from the CRS review of state APSRs are discussed in Appendix B.

CONCLUDING THOUGHTS

The findings from the state plans raise policy issues that may be relevant to Congress as it considers the next steps in oversight of psychotropic use among children in foster care. These issues include the use of medical homes and electronic health records to improve oversight of psychotropic medications, and the role of Medicaid in improving screenings and services for children in care with mental health needs. Other potential considerations are the involvement of children and youth in their mental health care and the extent to which states should report to HHS on their oversight policies.

Health Homes or Medical Homes

Children in foster care often lack consistent adults in their lives due to changes in living situations that result in new caregivers and possibly new caseworkers and health care providers. This may mean that no adult is fully aware of a child's current or prior mental health diagnoses or treatments, which creates an additional challenge in trying to identify and provide for a child's mental health needs. The concept of a "health home" or "medical home" is one way to address this challenge.

A "health home" is a strategy for helping people with chronic conditions, including mental health conditions, better manage those conditions through the provision of integrated services.[94] A health home can be a single person or a team of people that have access to the same information about a client or patient and coordinate treatment based on that information. In addition to addressing a person's physical and mental health conditions, health homes are meant to provide connections to community care services and supports, social services, and family services. Section 2703 of the Affordable Care Act, which enacted health care reforms, provides states with the option to cover health home services under Medicaid for eligible beneficiaries with target chronic conditions identified by each state. CMS has approved Medicaid state plan amendments for 12 states that have established health homes to coordinate care for these beneficiaries.[95] In guidance about the development of protocols for the appropriate use and monitoring of psychotropic medications, ACF indicates that state plans for ongoing oversight and coordination of health care services for children in foster care can incorporate a medical home for these children. Specifically, the plan must describe how states will "ensure a coordinated strategy to identify and respond to the health care needs of children in foster care placements ... and provide for continuity of health care services, which may include establishing a 'medical home' for children who are in foster care."[96] It is unclear the extent to which states in general are establishing health or medical homes for children in care under the authority of the Affordable Care Act or otherwise, though some states appear to have taken steps to do so.[97]

Electronic Health Records

One of the ways that health homes provide integrated services is by ensuring that all members of an individual's health home team have access to the same information. An important mechanism for providing that access is electronic health records (EHRs). The use of electronic health records has the potential to greatly improve information sharing among the stakeholders responsible for serving children in foster care. Separately from the protocols related to the oversight of the use of psychotropic medications, HHS instructed states to report in their state plans on "How medical information will be updated and appropriately shared, which may include developing and implementing an electronic health record."[98] The enhanced information sharing afforded by electronic health records could potentially improve the accuracy and efficacy of medical diagnoses and treatments, and provide easier access to data on the use of psychotropic medications for children in care.[99]

Existing federal health care law may be relevant to this issue. The Health Information Technology for Economic and Clinical Health Act, which was passed as part of the American Recovery and Reinvestment Act of 2009 (HITECH Act, P.L. 111-5), promotes the adoption of health information technology for the electronic sharing of clinical data through incentives and, in some cases, penalties.[100]

Medicaid

Most children in foster care receive medical care through the Medicaid program. As such, child welfare agencies, via the health care plans they provide children, would presumably be subject to or would have to incorporate or mirror Medicaid guidelines and policies in a wide range of areas, including the monitoring of psychotropic medications. The law requires that states must develop their health care oversight and coordination plan with the state Medicaid agency, among other stakeholders. Some states discussed how certain features of the Medicaid program—namely, Early and Periodic Screening, Diagnosis, and Treatment (EPSDT) services and the Drug Utilization Review (DUR)—are used to diagnose and respond to children in foster care with mental health needs. Nonetheless, HHS did not specifically request, and states generally did not address, how child welfare policies regarding oversight of psychotropic medications are connected to or comply with Medicaid policies.

Early and Periodic Screening, Diagnosis, and Treatment (EPSDT)

The EPSDT program is a required benefit for all children under age 21 who are covered by Medicaid. The program covers health screenings and services, including assessments of each child's physical and mental health development; laboratory tests (including lead blood level assessment); appropriate immunizations; health education; and vision, dental, and hearing services. The EPSDT program is intended to make health care services available and assist eligible children and their families in effectively using health care resources.[101]

However, it is unclear from the APSRs whether all states actually provide the screenings part of the program and include mental health as a component of these screenings. A 2010 report by the HHS Office of Inspector General (OIG) found that many Medicaid-eligible children did not receive all the EPSDT services, and this is consistent with earlier studies by the HHS OIG showing inconsistent receipt of basic health care services for children in foster care.[102] CMS has taken steps to work with states to promote access to mental health services for children through EPSDT, such as by forming a national EPSDT workgroup and issuing guidance to help inform states about resources available to help meet the mental health (and substance abuse) needs of children through EPSDT.[103] In conducting oversight on the use of psychotropic medication by children in care, Congress may choose to examine the extent to which these children in particular are receiving EPSDT services, and the extent to which mental health screenings and services are provided for this population.[104]

Drug Utilization Review

The Medicaid Drug Utilization Review (DUR) Program is a process through which state Medicaid agencies electronically monitor prescription drug claims to identify problems such as polypharmacy (the use of multiple medications at one time), incorrect dosage, or potential adverse drug interactions and analyze claims data to identify fraud or abuse. CMS requires all states to have DUR programs in place and to report annually on their state's pharmacy program operations, including the monitoring of prescription drugs.[105] DURs could be useful for the child welfare population because of the potential to flag the issues outlined previously. A small number of states provided information in their plans about how they are using their DURs to monitor oversight generally of children enrolled in Medicaid, including foster children. Still, it is unclear how most states coordinate prescription drug monitoring efforts with the state DUR program.

Youth Engagement

States were not specifically asked to discuss how they engage children and youth in oversight of psychotropic medications; however, this appears to be somewhat implied under the second protocol, which addresses informed and shared decision-making (consent and assent) and methods for ongoing communication between various stakeholders, including the child. HHS has identified "youth engagement and empowerment" as a component of strengthening management of psychotropic medications.[106] Few states described the involvement of young people in making decisions about their mental health treatment or taking psychotropic medications. Eleven states reported involving children in the consent process, and one state specifically mentioned that it had plans to provide information to foster children about the use of psychotropic medications.

With support from SAMHSA, AACAP developed guidance for child and adolescent psychiatrists to communicate and partner with youth about their treatment.[107] Congress might choose to examine whether such guidance might be useful for states to distribute to stakeholders involved in the mental health care of children in foster care.

Reporting on Oversight

In its program instructions, HHS directed states to provide fairly detailed information beyond basic information about "the oversight of prescription medicines, including protocols for the appropriate use and monitoring of psychotropic medications." HHS specifically requested information about the methods and policies states implement to coordinate screenings and assessment to identify mental health needs, availability of mental health expertise to consult with the child welfare agencies, and monitoring of medications for individuals in foster care and all children in care generally, among other items. Given the breadth of information requested and provided, an issue might be whether more specific and uniform information should be gathered from states. For example, Congress could request that HHS provide a summary of information about certain aspects of oversight and define terms that are relevant to this oversight (e.g., psychotropics, medication, screening, board-certified or board-eligible psychiatrist, training) to better capture uniform information across states. Still, more narrowly focused reporting may not necessarily yield responses that can be easily synthesized across states.

APPENDIX A. USE OF PSYCHOTROPICS AMONG CHILDREN IN FAMILIES INVESTIGATED FOR ABUSE OR NEGLECT

The National Survey of Child and Adolescent Wellbeing (NSCAW) II looked at rates of psychotropic medication use among a sample of children (5,873) who came into contact with the child welfare agency because of an investigation of child abuse or neglect in their families. Initial (baseline) survey data were collected in 2008-2009 approximately four to six months after that investigation. With regard to use of psychotropic medication, data cover children who at the time of the initial survey were at least 18 months of age and up to 17 years old. A follow-up survey looked at psychotropic medication use among these same children at approximately 18 months after the investigation of abuse or neglect, and a third survey looked at those children at 36 months following the investigation. (Some of the children followed had reached age 18 or older by the second or third collection of data.)

Table A-1 shows psychotropic medication use by age, and whether or not the child was in a foster care setting for the initial survey and for the follow-up at 18 months and 36 months. For purposes of this analysis, a foster care setting includes children who were placed in a non-relative foster family home, children placed with kin on a formal basis, and children placed in a group or residential setting. By contrast, children included in the "in home" category includes children living with their biological or adoptive parents, as well as children who were in informal kinship care settings.

Table A-1. Current Use of Psychotropic Medication Among Children in Families Investigated for Child Abuse or Neglect

Percentages based on caregiver report at time of interview or youth self-report for those 18 or older

Age at Time of Survey and Placement Status of Children	Initial Survey	18-Month Follow-Up	36-Month Follow-Up
TOTAL (18 months or older)			
Foster Care	15.9%	23.1%a	32.8%a
In-home	11.6%	11.0%	12.9%
Ages 18 months to 5 yearsb			
Foster Care	3.7%	1.5%	8.8%
In-home	1.4%	1.6%	1.6%
Ages 6-10 years			
Foster Care	21.3%	37.0%a	27.6%
In-home	19.5%	19.2%	16.1%
Ages 11-17 years			
Foster Care	26.8%	39.9%a	47.0%a
In-home	15.7%	13.8%	16.5%
Age 18 or older			
Include all youth age 18 or older regardless of where they lived.	NA	7.9%	11.3%

Source: Congressional Research Service, based on data from NSCAW II as received from the U.S. Department of Health and Human Services, Administration for Children and Families, Office of Planning Research and Evaluation (OPRE), January 2014.

Note: Children in the sample were not necessarily in foster care for the entire 18- or 36-month period. They may have entered and re-entered care during this time, or they could have entered care after a subsequent investigation. Children in foster care include those who were living in a non-relative foster family home, formal kinship care, or a group home/residential program. Those shown as living "in-home" were those who remained with their biological or adoptive parents or those who were living informally in kinship care.

[a] Indicates that children in this group of foster care children were significantly more likely to be taking psychotropic medication than the comparable group of children who were living in their own homes during the same point in time.

[b] The overall NSCAW sample included children as young as two months at the beginning of the study. The data on psychotropic use includes children in the sample who were 18 months and older. Some children in the sample were not yet 18 months old at the initial survey, and later aged into the sample at the 18-month follow-up. This led to an increase in the overall number of children in the sample at 18 months and 36 months.

Statistical Significance

The percentage differences shown by the initial survey in use of psychotropic medication (between children in foster care and those who were not in foster care) were not statistically significant overall or for any specific age group shown in Table A-1. However, the differences shown for these groups at the 18-month and 36-month follow-up were statistically significant, with children in foster care more likely to be using psychotropic medications.

For children under age 6, there was no statistical significance found in the percentage differences shown for children in foster care versus those living at home in any of the surveys (initial, 18- month or 36-month). For children ages 6 to 10, the percentage difference shown between the in-home and foster care groups at the 18-month follow-up was found to be statistically significant but not those shown at the initial survey or at the 36-month follow-up. For children ages 11 through 17 years, there was not statistical significance found between the in-home and foster care groups at the initial survey but the differences shown at the 18-month and 36-month follow-up were significant.

APPENDIX B. FINDINGS FROM CRS REVIEW OF STATE OVERSIGHT OF PSYCHOTROPIC MEDICATION

Beginning with FY2012, the U.S. Department of Health and Human Services (HHS) has required states to provide specific information on state protocols for use of psychotropic medication. States were required to provide this information in their Annual Progress and Services Report (APSR), which is part of the documentation states must submit to receive funding under the Stephanie Tubbs Jones Child Welfare Services Program (Child Welfare Services Program). This documentation is known as the Child and Family Services Plan.

HHS provided CRS with the 2012 APSRs between March and September of 2013. The 2012 APSR includes information about state procedures that were in place at least through the submission deadline of June 2012.[108] The review examined portions of the APSR that addressed the five oversight areas, or protocols: (1) mental health evaluations and treatment planning; (2) consent, assent, and ongoing communication; (3) psychotropic medication monitoring; (4) availability of "board-certified" child and adolescent psychiatrists; and (5) education and training about psychotropics.

follow-up period (every six months, biannually, etc.) while others indicated that the screenings/assessments are conducted periodically.

Treatment Planning

As part of the first protocol, states were asked to discuss their efforts at carrying out treatment planning for children's mental health needs. Eighteen states provided information about steps they take in responding to health care screenings and assessments. Some states indicated that children are referred for additional evaluations, while other states indicated that children are referred for or are provided services. Services were sometimes specified, and included substance abuse services, inpatient psychiatric care, and other mental health interventions. Two states mentioned that psychiatric medications may be appropriate to respond to children's mental health needs. Further, two states indicated that information from the screening or assessment is incorporated into the child's case plan.

Trauma

As specified above, 10 states specified that they had a trauma screening tool only, or a trauma screening tool in addition to the mental health screening tool. Generally, states did not define trauma except to say that children may be traumatized by certain events. Two states addressed how children in care who have experienced trauma receive treatment, such as through trauma treatment centers and community mental health centers. Nine states indicated that they have plans to develop trauma screening tools or to implement such tools soon.

Protocol 2: Informed and Shared Decision-Making (Consent and Assent) and Methods for Ongoing Communication

For protocol 2, states were asked to describe any written policies that address "informed and shared decision-making (consent and assent) and methods for ongoing communication between the prescriber, the child, his/her caregivers, other healthcare providers, the child welfare worker, and other key stakeholders." *Consent* and *assent* were not defined in the program instructions but these terms are commonly used in medical literature.[112] In the context of medical care and research, *consent*, or *informed consent*, refers to the process through which a person receives information about a particular health condition and treatment options, including benefits and risks; understands that information; and agrees to receive one (or more) of the treatment options. The research literature stated that *consent* has legal force and generally involves obtaining a signature from the person who will receive treatment. *Assent* is similar to *consent* in that it involves informing a person about a health condition and treatment options and obtaining agreement from the person to pursue a particular treatment. However, *assent* does not have legal force. *Assent* generally refers to agreement obtained from a minor or from an adult who does not have the legal capacity to provide *consent*.

More than half of the states (34 of 52) provided some information about this protocol in their APSR. States addressed various aspects of consent, assent, and communication, including

- who provides consent or assent;
- pre-authorization processes;
- communication during the consent process;
- who may prescribe psychotropic medications; and
- communication after a child has begun treatment with a psychotropic medication.

Who Provides Consent or Assent

States indicated that consent involves one or more of the following parties: a parent/legal guardian, the child, the child welfare agency, or a court/judge. These parties may be involved concurrently, their involvement may depend upon the child's legal status, and their involvement may be required or recommended. In Connecticut, for example, consent is obtained from the parent, legal guardian, or child welfare agency (depending on the child's legal status) and assent must be obtained from children age 14 or older. In Indiana, the parent, guardian, or custodian and the child welfare agency must give consent. Arizona recommends that the person from the home where the child is currently residing provide consent.

Of the states that provided information on this protocol, over half (18 of 34) reported that a *parent or legal guardian* is involved in providing consent, most often as the first or primary consenting authority. With regard to parental consent (versus that of a legal guardian), multiple states indicated that parental consent is not sought or is not required under one or more of the following circumstances: parental rights have been relinquished or terminated, a parent cannot be located or is not available, or a parent is unable to make a decision due to physical or mental impairment.

Eleven states reported involving *children* in the consent process. What this involvement looks like varies significantly from state to state. For example,

Connecticut and Alabama require assent or consent from children of a certain age in addition to consent from a parent or guardian. In New Mexico and Washington, children of a certain age have sole authority to consent to being treated with psychotropic medications. Other states, such as Florida and New Jersey, require or suggest that children be involved in discussions about the use of psychotropic medications.

Sixteen states reported that the *child welfare agency* is involved in some way in providing consent. In eight states, the child welfare agency provides consent in some or all instances where parental rights have been terminated or relinquished or a parent is not available. The consent may be provided by an agency director or commissioner, a caseworker or social worker, an agency medical director or nurse, or a special consent unit within the agency. In five states, the child welfare agency is the only consenting authority in some or all instances where psychotropics are prescribed. In three states, it appears that the child welfare agency and the parent or guardian must both provide consent.

Thirteen states reported that a *court or a judge* may be involved in authorizing the use of psychotropic medication for children in foster care. In 11 states, a court order is required when parental rights have been terminated or relinquished, when a parent is unavailable to provide consent, or when consent has been denied by a parent/guardian and/or child. California law requires judicial approval prior to the administration of psychotropic medications under any circumstances. Massachusetts requires judicial approval for treatment with psychotropics that are antipsychotics.

Two states take a slightly different approach to consent. In Nevada, a "Person Legally Responsible" (PLR) is designated as the only party who may provide consent for a child. The PLR could be a foster parent, an attorney, a relative of the child, an employee of the child welfare agency, or any other person who a court determines is qualified. Texas law requires that each child in state child welfare conservatorship have a designated "medical consenter" who makes medical decisions for the child. Typically the medical consenter is the child's caregiver or a caseworker, though it could be another party.

Eight states noted in their APSR that psychotropic medications may be administered without consent in an emergency where a child may harm himself/herself or others and the medication is deemed to be the only way or the best way to treat the child. In Tennessee, however, the emergency use of psychotropic medication is allowed only for children in hospital facilities or facilities designated as psychiatric residential treatment facilities per federal guidelines.

Pre-Authorization

Some states reported requiring a pre-authorization process for the use of psychotropic medications, in addition to consent or as a part of consent. The process varies from state to state, but it typically requires the prescriber to submit a request with details about the child, the diagnosis, and the medication to a board, committee, team, or other designated authority that must approve the request before treatment can begin. Eight states reported requiring pre-authorization for the use of certain psychotropic medications or for the use of psychotropics with children under a certain age. Three additional states reported having plans to implement a pre-authorization process.

Information Sharing during the Consent Process

Fourteen states provided a description of the information that is shared among stakeholders (parents/legal guardians, child, child welfare agency, health care providers) as part of the consent process. Most of these states described communication where a health care provider or child welfare agency employee provides information to the parent/legal guardian and/or child. Some states indicated that the sharing of certain information is required as part of the consent process, while others indicated that it is suggested or recommended. The types of information most frequently mentioned in the APSRs include the following:

- nature of diagnosis,
- name of medication and dosage,
- benefit(s) or expected result(s),
- potential side effects,
- long-term and short-term risks, and
- alternative therapies.

Who May Prescribe Psychotropic Medications

When describing who may prescribe psychotropic medications, most states used the term "provider" or "prescriber." Eight states provided more specific descriptions about who may or who should prescribe, such as a licensed or licensed and certified physician; a board certified or board eligible specialist in psychiatry, neurodevelopmental pediatrics, or pediatric neurology; a qualified psychiatrist; a psychiatric nurse practitioner; or a developmental pediatrician. Some states indicated that who may prescribe depends upon the type of medication. For example, Arizona explained that "[o]nly physicians (psychiatrists), physician assistants, or nurse practitioners credentialed and licensed by the Tribal and Regional Behavioral Health Authorities may prescribe psychotropic medications. A child's primary care physician may write prescriptions for patients with minor depression, anxiety disorders and treatment of ADHD without co-morbidity."

Methods for Ongoing Communication

For the purposes of this report, "methods for ongoing communication" is interpreted as referring to communication that takes place after a child has begun treatment with a psychotropic medication, as distinguished from communication and information sharing that takes place as part of the consent process. Twenty-two states provided some information about methods for ongoing communication, and there was a great deal of variation among the descriptions. Notably, aspects of "ongoing communication" are also closely tied to monitoring issues, which are addressed in the next section of the report.

Some of the specific mechanisms that states cited as facilitating communication include databases, a child's medical passport or medical record, caseworker visits with a child and his/her caregiver family, phone calls between stakeholders, child and family team meetings, websites, email messages, and reports or forms. The types of information shared as a part of ongoing communication include medication details, treatment notes, medical histories, medication benefits or side effects, changes in medication (type, dosage, frequency, stopping use), medication administration, agency policies and procedures, and contact information for stakeholders. The people mentioned in the APSRs as being involved in ongoing communication include representatives of child welfare agencies (caseworker, social worker, supervisor, etc.), health care providers (primary care physician, nurse, prescribing provider), the child or client, and the caregivers or foster parents. The flow of information among these people was most often described as going from a child welfare agency representative or health care provider to the child and/or caregivers.

Protocol 3: Effective Medication Monitoring at the Client and Agency Level

For protocol 3, states were asked to describe any written policies related to effective medication monitoring at both the client and agency level. The program instructions did not provide any further detail about what was meant by "medication monitoring" or client-level versus agency-level monitoring. Based on the CRS review of APSRs, "medication monitoring at the client level" seems to encompass monitoring of how a specific medication affects the client as well as monitoring of a client's overall medication treatment plan. "Medication monitoring at the agency level" seems to refer primarily, though not exclusively, to the monitoring of prescribing patterns across a child welfare agency's entire caseload.

Thirty-eight states provided some information about this protocol. Of those 38, 13 provided general or limited information and the other 25 provided broader or more detailed information. States addressed a number of different aspects of monitoring, including what is being monitored, who is doing the monitoring, and mechanisms used to conduct monitoring. The following two subsections look at these aspects, first in relation to client-level monitoring and then agency-level monitoring.

Client-Level Monitoring

Thirty-six states provided information about medication monitoring at the client level. States described monitoring both the child and the child's prescriptions. Monitoring of the child is primarily focused on determining how the medication is affecting him/her. Specifically, states most frequently mentioned monitoring for side effects (15 states) and whether targeted symptoms have improved, remained the same, or deteriorated (11 states). States also mentioned monitoring of specific physiologic measures such as a child's weight, height, body mass index, blood pressure, heart rate, respiratory rate, glucose levels, and lipid levels, as well as being alert to potential drug interactions, and identifying any issues that the child or caregiver might have with administering medications.

Twenty-five states provided information about who conducts the monitoring of individual children. These include health care providers (prescriber, nurse, physician, medical director, psychiatrist, pharmacist); child welfare agency staff (caseworker, supervisor, manager); third-parties (medical consultant, medical expert, independent reviewer); caregivers (foster parent, legal guardian); and the individual child. Some states described a team that is involved with monitoring, which can be a combination of individuals from one or more of the previous categories.

Thirty-six states described mechanisms used to monitor how medication is affecting an individual child. These include conversations between the child and caregiver and between the child, caregiver, and caseworker; logs maintained by the caregiver; medical check-ups; medical records; databases;

and team meetings. Fourteen states mentioned the frequency of visits or check-ups with either a caseworker or a health care provider. Twelve of the fourteen states gave a specific time frame such as "at least once a month" or "one to two weeks after starting the medication," while two stated that the frequency of follow-up appointments would vary by client depending on factors such as the medication, the diagnosis, and how the child was responding.

States explained that the monitoring of a child's prescriptions involved establishing guidelines for prescribers to follow and then identifying red flags in prescriptions that could necessitate further review of the child's diagnosis and treatment plan. The following were identified by states as possible sources of concern in a prescription: polypharmacy[113] (12 states), use of certain medications with children under certain ages (9 states), dosage exceeding what is recommended (6 states), potential adverse drug interactions (3 states), and a mismatch between prescription and diagnosis (3 states). According to states, the parties involved in the monitoring of a child's prescription could include pharmacists, caseworkers, health care providers other than the prescriber, third-party reviewers or consultants, and, somewhat indirectly, committees or review boards. Committees or review boards typically conduct agency-level monitoring (see the next section), but their work can identify particular cases that require further review, which in turn could lead to changes in an individual child's treatment plan. States described a number of different mechanisms that could be used to monitor a child's prescriptions. These include review of a child's medical record; tracking prescriptions in databases; committee or review board meetings within the child welfare agency or across state agencies (see the next section); and a pre-authorization process for medication consent (as discussed under protocol 2).

Agency-Level Monitoring

Twenty-five states provided information about medication monitoring at the agency level. Ten of the 25 provided general or limited information and 15 provided more specific and/or broader information. In terms of what is being monitored, 18 states referred to monitoring prescribing patterns or something similar. Other terms used include drug utilization patterns, prescribing trends, prescribing practices, and compliance with prescribing guidelines. Some states cited specific aspects of prescribing patterns or trends that they track such as rates of polypharmacy and co-pharmacy (Illinois) or types of medications and the number of children receiving medications (Montana).

States also described other aspects of medication monitoring such as tracking consent request outcomes (Illinois and Connecticut), the use of emergency medications (Illinois), and FDA medication cautions (Utah). Six states specifically mentioned that agency-level monitoring is used to identify prescriptions or prescribers that do not comply with established guidelines. States identified a number of different parties that could be involved in conducting agency-level monitoring. Eleven states indicated that the child welfare agency is responsible for agency-level monitoring. Of these 11 states, 3 identified a specific subunit within the agency that handles monitoring. For example, Illinois has a Centralized Psychopharmacology Consent Program through which board certified child psychiatric consultants provide an independent medication review of all psychotropic medication consent requests. Three of the 11 states indicated that the overall health care program for children in foster care is responsible for agency-level monitoring. Three states identified individuals involved in agency-level monitoring, such as a chief psychiatrist, chief medical officer, or child psychiatry consultant. Seven states described special committees or review boards that are involved in agency-level monitoring (for example, the Psychopharmacology Advisory Committee in Kansas). These committees or review boards may include members from the child welfare agency as well as other state agencies and outside consultants. In some states, these entities originate in the state Medicaid program as a part of required Drug Utilization Review Programs.[114]

States described using a number of different mechanisms to conduct agency-level monitoring. Seven states referred to reports containing aggregate and/or individual case information over a specific period of time. Three of these seven states specifically mentioned that the reports were based on claims data. Eight states indicated that claims data was a source of information used in monitoring, and five states specifically mentioned using Medicaid claims or payment data. Four states reported that meetings of monitoring bodies are used to review and discuss the use of psychotropic medications. For example, Iowa's Drug Utilization Review Board reviews 300 member profiles at each of its six annual meetings.

Protocol 4: Availability of Mental Health Expertise and Consultation

The fourth protocol asked states to describe policies related to the "availability of mental health expertise and consultation regarding both consent and monitoring issues by a board-certified or board-eligible child and adolescent psychiatrist (at both the agency and individual case level)." The

2012 HHS program instructions do not define "board-certified or board-eligible child and adolescent psychiatrist." According to the American Board of Psychiatry and Neurology (ABPN), a nonprofit medical organization that oversees doctor certification in psychiatry and neurology, a board certified psychiatrist is one who has completed the required training in a specialty of psychiatry and has passed an exam administered by the ABPN.[115] The term "board-eligible" refers to a doctor who has met the requirements to stand for a certification exam, but who has not yet taken the exam.[116]

Seven states specifically reported having access to "board-certified" or "board-eligible" child and adolescent psychiatrists for consultation or review related to the use of psychotropic medications. Thirteen states reported having access to a psychiatrist, a child/adolescent psychiatrist, or a psychiatric consultation service but did not specifically use the term "board-certified" or "board-eligible." (Nevada falls into both groups of states as child welfare services in the state are provided by three entities whose policies are not identical.) States did not provide a great deal of detail on this protocol, and most of the information addresses the availability of mental health expertise for individual children rather than for the child welfare agency overall.

Nine states described in general terms the role of the psychiatrist or psychiatric consultation service for an individual child. For example, South Dakota explained that the child welfare agency is able to consult with board certified child psychiatrists and psychiatric nurses from the South Dakota Foundation of Medical Providers and Peer Review Organization and child psychiatrists contracting with Psychiatric Residential Care providers.

Several states described more specific ways that psychiatrists are involved in consent and monitoring for individual children. Florida, Oklahoma, and Wyoming have hotlines through which primary care providers or, in the case of Oklahoma, child welfare agency staff, can obtain a psychiatric consultation. Connecticut, Hawaii, and Illinois describe in-person consultations with psychiatrists on specific cases. These consultations could be conducted with prescribers, child welfare agency staff, or other stakeholders. Illinois and Connecticut have centralized medication consent processes, and board certified child psychiatrists play a role in the approval of consent requests. Four states involve psychiatrists in reviewing specific cases if one or more red flags have been triggered by a prescription.

Only three states described how psychiatrists provide consultation at the agency level. In Connecticut, a board-certified child psychiatrist serves as Chief of Psychiatry for the child welfare agency and is responsible for policy development and supervision of the Centralized Medication Consent Unit. In

Michigan, the child welfare agency has a board-certified child and adolescent psychiatrist who provides education and outreach to physicians and health liaison officers throughout the state. New Jersey's child welfare agency has a child and adolescent psychiatrist who "provides leadership around quality assurance efforts ... and ongoing efforts to strengthen the agency's psychotropic medication policy."

Protocol 5: Mechanisms for Accessing and Sharing Accurate and Up-to-Date Information and Educational Materials

States were further asked to provide information about mechanisms for accessing and sharing mental health and trauma-related information with clinicians, child welfare staff, and consumers. Thirty-five states provided a response to this protocol; 17 states did not. The APSR guidance does not define what these mechanisms entail, and states generally responded that such mechanisms include training, publications, and other materials about psychotropic medications. States indicated that training is available for child welfare staff; clinicians; and other child welfare stakeholders, including foster parents, staff at residential facilities, juvenile justice agency staff, and children's advocacy groups. "Consumers" is not defined in the APSR guidance; however, it appears to refer to the children who are prescribed psychotropic medications. States generally did not indicate that information and educational materials are provided to children in care, although one state (Hawaii) indicated that it had plans to provide information to foster children.

Information for Child Welfare Staff

Twenty-six states provided information about training that is provided or will be provided to child welfare staff about policies on psychotropic medications and/or treatment planning, including on trauma-informed interventions. Some states provide or plan to provide training to all child welfare workers, new child welfare workers only, supervisors, or selected child welfare staff. For example, Connecticut stated that it provides training for all new workers regarding psychotropic medication policies. In addition, the training for area child welfare directors and social workers includes information about prescribing trends for children in care. South Carolina indicated that one area of the state was in the process of carrying out a pilot program to identify protocols for psychotropic monitoring. Training was provided for one and a half days to social workers, supervisors, and a regional clinical coordinator in the pilot area on the use of psychotropic medications. Twelve states specifically mentioned that training addressed trauma, including treatment of trauma.

Some states provided information about which individuals or entities conduct the training for workers: the state child welfare agency, including health personnel or a health unit within the child welfare agency; a state health or mental health agency; mental health consultants; or an outside entity that specializes in treatment of trauma (Chadwick Center for Children & Families at Rady Children's Hospital in San Diego, Children's Trauma Assessment Center at Western Michigan University, and Kennedy Krieger Family Center in Baltimore). Texas discussed that an online training is available for child welfare staff and other stakeholders that is accessible via the state child welfare agency website. Louisiana indicated that it had plans to adapt this online training for its staff and other stakeholders.

A small number of states provided information about the publications and materials that have been provided to child welfare staff about oversight of psychotropic medications, including

- an online child welfare manual about informed consent and best practices for use of psychotropic medications;
- materials for child family team meetings that involve children who are prescribed psychotropic medications;
- the AACAP guidelines;
- state child welfare agency guidelines (which reference the AACAP guidelines) about oversight of psychotropic medications; and
- policy transmittals about psychotropics.

Information for Clinicians

Nine states discussed the information that is disseminated or will be disseminated to clinicians about child welfare or other state policies about psychotropic medication use by children in foster care. States indicated that clinicians receive or will receive information about the child welfare agency's system for prescribing psychotropic medications for children in foster care, including the consent process and oversight; changes in state child welfare policies on prescribing medications; where state policies are available online; best practice guidelines for prescribing; new label information on psychotropics and warnings by the Food and Drug Administration (FDA); and data on children in foster care who are prescribed psychotropic drugs. According to states, this information has been or will be conveyed via phone calls between child welfare staff and clinicians, state Medicaid program publications, faxed forms, the child welfare agency website, and teleconference.

Information for Other Stakeholders

Finally, 12 states indicated that they provided information to other child welfare stakeholders about policies on psychotropic drug use for children in foster care, or had plans to do so. These other stakeholders included foster parents, staff at group homes and other group-care settings for children in care; biological parents; child-serving community organizations; and other state agencies and individuals that may interact with children in foster care. Hawaii indicated that it plans to provide information and awareness about the dangers of the use of psychotropic medications to children in foster care, judges, lawyers, teachers, guardians ad litem, court appointed special advocates, and the general public. States explained that these other stakeholders received information through a written guide, an online training, training for state agencies or child-serving organizations, and foster parent training. In some cases, the training focused on trauma and treatments for trauma.

End Notes

[1] Psychotropic drug classes include those for attention deficit hyperactivity disorder (ADHD), antianxiety, antidepressants, antipsychotics, hypnotics, and mood stabilizers. For further information, see Table 1 of U.S. Government Accountability Office (GAO), *Foster Children: HHS Guidance Could Help States Improve Oversight of Psychotropic Prescriptions*, GAO-12-201, December 2011, http://gao.gov/products/GAO-12-201. (Hereinafter, GAO, *Foster Children: HHS Guidance Could Help States Improve Oversight of Psychotropic Prescriptions*.)

[2] A small percentage of children nationwide enter foster care via "voluntary placement agreements." In these situations a parent or guardian signs over certain care and placement responsibility to the state child welfare agency and, after six months, a judge may be asked to determine if this placement continues to be in the "best interest" of the child.

[3] "Neglect" was associated with removal and entry to foster care of close to two-thirds (65%) of children entering care at age 12 or younger and 36% of those entering at ages 13 through 17. By contrast, a "child's behavior problem" was associated with removal of less than 3% of children entering care at age 12 or younger and close to 45% of those children entering care at age 13 through 17 years of age. Based on state data reported via the Adoption and Foster Care Analysis Reporting System (AFCARS) as of July 2014 and provided to CRS by the U.S. Department of Health and Human Services (HHS), Administration for Children

and Families (ACF), Administration for Children, Youth and Families (ACYF), Children's Bureau. Each child could have one or more reasons associated with his or her removal from the home and entry to foster care. For more information, see U.S. House of Representatives, Committee on Ways and Means, *2014 Green Book,* Chapter 11, "Child Welfare," "Additional Tables and Figures," Tables 11-7 and 11-7A.

[4] HHS, ACF, ACYF, Children's Bureau, *Trends in Foster Care and Adoption: FFY 2002-FFY 2013,* based on AFCARS data reported by state as of July 21, 2014.

[5] John Landsverk, Barbara Burns, Leyla Stambaugh, and Jennifer A. Rolls Reutz, *Mental Health Care for Children and Adolescents in Foster Care: Review of Research Literature,* prepared for Casey Family Programs, February 2006.

[6] John Stirling Jr., and Lisa Amaya-Jackson, "Understanding the Behavioral and Emotional Consequences of Child Abuse," American Academy of Pediatrics Clinical Report, *Pediatrics,* vol. 122, no. 3, September 2008, pp. 667-673. Jun-Qing Liu, "Mental Health Service Access Among Children and Adolescents Involved with Child Welfare Services," Dissertation, University of Albany, State University of New York, 2011.

[7] Heather Ringeisen et al., *NSCAW II Baseline Report: Children's Services,* Final Report, RTI International for HHS, ACF, Office of Planning, Research and Evaluation, November 2011, p. 33. This report shows risk at the lower end (43% or 61%, depending on placement setting) and is based on survey data collected 4 to 6 months after the investigation of child abuse and neglect that brought the child to the attention of the child welfare agency. (Hereinafter, Heather Ringeisen et al., *NSCAW II Baseline Report: Children's Services.*) Cecilia Casanueva et al., *NSCAW II Wave 2 Report: Children's Services,* Final Report, RTI International for HHS, ACF, Office of Planning, Research and Evaluation, July 2012, pp. 9-11. This report shows risk at the higher end of range (45% or 70% depending on placement setting) and is based on survey data collected regarding the same group of children circa 18 months after the investigation of child abuse and neglect that brought the child to the attention of the child welfare agency. (Hereinafter, Cecilia Casanueva et al., *NSCAW II Wave 2 Report: Children's Services.*) The risk of a behavioral/emotional problem was defined as scores in the clinical range on any of the following standardized measures: Internalizing, Externalizing or Total Problems scales of the Child Behavior Checklist, Youth Self Report (YSR), or the Teacher Report Form (TRF); the Child Depression Inventory (CDI), or the Post Traumatic Stress section Intrusive Experiences and Disassociation subscales of the Trauma Symptoms Checklist. These estimates are based on participants' perceptions of symptoms rather than direct clinical diagnoses.

[8] Cecilia Casanueva et al., *NSCAW II Wave 2 Report: Children's Services,* pp. 9-11. Exact comparable data for the general population are not available. Estimates cited in this report are based on national surveys (conducted between 2001 and 2007) that used somewhat different measures for determining emotional and behavioral concerns among children ages 2 to 17 or ages 4 to 17.

[9] For purposes of Medicaid eligibility "foster care" status extends to some (but not all) children in foster care, most children who are adopted from foster care, and certain children who have aged out of foster care. For further information, "Limitations on Understanding Medicaid Spending for Foster Care Children," in CRS Report R42378, *Child Welfare: Health Care Needs of Children in Foster Care and Related Federal Issues,* by Emilie Stoltzfus et al.

[10] David Rubin et al., "Interstate Variation in Trends of Psychotropic Medication Use Among Medicaid-enrolled Children in Foster Care," *Child and Youth Services Review,* vol. 34, no. 8 (2012), p. 1492. (Hereinafter, David Rubin et al., "Interstate Variation in Trends of Psychotropic Medication Use Among Medicaid-enrolled Children in Foster Care.") This

study counted a child as in foster care if, in a given year (FY2002-FY2007), the child had at least one month of Medicaid eligibility under the "foster care child" eligibility pathway.

[11] Mark Olfson et al., "National Trends in the Mental Health Care of Children, Adolescents, and Adults by Office-Based Physicians," The *Journal of the American Medical Association,* vol. 71, no. 1, January 2014. (Hereinafter Mark Olfson et al., "National Trends in the Mental Health Care of Children, Adolescents, and Adults by Office-Based Physicians.")

[12] The report does not define these or other mental conditions that have been studied. The American Psychiatric Association's Diagnostic and Statistical Manual (DSM) is the standard classification of mental disorders used by mental health professionals, and defines these terms. For further information, see American Psychiatric Association, "DSM," http://www.psychiatry.org/practice/dsm.

[13] Medicaid is a means-tested program available primarily to children whose families meet certain income eligibility tests. Children in foster care may qualify for Medicaid through a federal eligibility pathway specifically for them. For further information, see CRS Report R42378, *Child Welfare: Health Care Needs of Children in Foster Care and Related Federal Issues*, by Emilie Stoltzfus et al., Child Welfare: Health Care Needs of Children in Foster Care and Related Federal Issues.

[14] David Rubin et al., "Interstate Variation in Trends of Psychotropic Medication Use Among Medicaid-enrolled Children in Foster Care."

[15] Ramesh Raghavan et al., "A Preliminary Analysis of the Receipt of Mental Health Services Consistent with National Standards Among Children in the Child Welfare System," *American Journal of Public Health,* vol. 100, no. 4 (April 2010).

[16] CRS Report R42378, *Child Welfare: Health Care Needs of Children in Foster Care and Related Federal Issues*, by Emilie Stoltzfus et al.

[17] HHS, ACF, ACYF, Children's Bureau, "Promoting Social and Emotional Well-Being for Children and Youth Receiving Child Welfare Services," Information Memorandum ACYF-CB-IM-12-04, April 17, 2012, http://www.acf.hhs.gov/sites/default/files/cb/im1204.pdf. (Hereinafter, HHS, ACF, ACYF, Children's Bureau, "Promoting Social and Emotional Well-Being for Children and Youth Receiving Child Welfare Services." April 2012). See also HHS, ACF, Centers for Medicare and Medicaid Services (CMS), Substance Abuse and Mental Health Services Administration (SAMHSA), "Dear State Director," July 11, 2013, http://medicaid.gov/Federal-PolicyGuidance/Downloads/SMD-13-07-11.pdf.   (Hereinafter U.S. Department of Health and Human Services, ACF, CMS, and SAMHSA, "Dear State Director," July 2013.)

[18] HHS, ACF, CMS, SAMHSA, "Dear State Director," July 2013.

[19] Christine M. Litschge, Michael G. Vaughn, Cynthia McCrea, "The Empirical Status of Treatments for Children and Youth with Conduct Problems: An Overview of Meta-Analytical Studies," *Research on Social Work Practice*, vol. 20, no. 1 (2010).

[20] Holly R. Wethington et al., "The Effectiveness of Interventions to Reduce Psychological Harm from Traumatic Events Among Children and Adolescents: A Systematic Review," *American Journal of Preventative Medicine,* vol. 35, no. 3 (2008).

[21] Leyla F. Stambaugh et al., *Psychotropic Medication Use by Children in Child Welfare*, HHS, ACF, Office of Planning, Research, and Evaluation (OPRE), National Survey of Child and Adolescent Well-Being II Report. No. 17, 2012, http://www.acf.hhs.gov/programs/opre/resource/nscaw-no-17-psychotropic-medication-use-by-children-in-childwelfare. (Hereinafter Leyla F. Stambaugh et al., *Psychotropic Medication Use by Children in Child Welfare.*)

[22] The Children's Hospital of Philadelphia, "New PolicyLab Research Expands Understanding of Psychoactive Medication Use Among Children in Foster Care," press release, April 30, 2012, http://www.chop.edu/news/psychoactive-drug-use-among-children-in-foster-care.html.

[23] Leyla F. Stambaugh et al., *Psychotropic Medication Use by Children in Child Welfare*.

[24] Barbara J. Burns et al., "Mental Health Needs and Access to Mental Health Services by Youths Involved with Child Welfare: A National Survey," *Journal of the American Academy of Child and Adolescent Psychiatry*, vol. 43, no. 8, 2004, pp. 960-970; Laurel K. Leslie et al., "Relationship Between Entry Into Child Welfare and Mental Health Service Use," *Psychiatric Services*, vol. 56, no. 8 (August 2005), p. 985.

[25] Leyla F. Stambaugh et al., *Psychotropic Medication Use by Children in Child Welfare*. Specialty mental health services include an outpatient drug or alcohol clinic, mental health or community health center, private mental health professional, in-home counseling or crisis services, treatment for emotional and substance abuse problems, therapeutic nursery, psychiatric unit in hospital, detox or inpatient unit, hospital medical inpatient unit, residential treatment center or group home, hospital emergency room for emotional and substance abuse problems, family doctor mental health service, and school-based mental health service.

[26] Based on data from NSCAW II as received from the U.S. Department of Health and Human Services, Administration for Children and Families, Office of Planning Research and Evaluation (OPRE), January 2014. For more information, see Appendix A.

[27] Leyla F. Stambaugh et al., *Psychotropic Medication Use by Children in Child Welfare*, p. 3. This prevalence is based on data from National Health Interview Survey, fielded in 2005 and 2006, and which looked at use of psychotropic drugs among children (ages 4 to 17 years) who were prescribed psychotropic drugs in the last 12 months.

[28] Ibid. See also GAO, *Foster Children: HHS Guidance Could Help States Improve Oversight of Psychotropic Prescriptions*.

[29] Kathleen R. Merikangas, et.al., "Medication Use in US Youth with Mental Disorders," *JAMA Pediatrics*, v. 167, no. 2 (2013), p. 141-148. This prevalence is based on national survey of general population of adolescents in the United States (National Comorbidity Survey Adolescent Supplement).

[30] Lynn A. Warner, Na Kyoung Song, and Kathleen J. Pottick, "Outpatient Psychotropic Medication Use in the U.S.: A Comparison Based on Foster Care Status," *Journal of Child and Family Studies*, December 10, 2013, vol. 23, no. 4, pp. 652-665. The study is the Client/Patient Sample Survey, carried out by HHS, Substance Abuse and Mental Health Services Administration (SAMHSA) and the Centers for Medicare and Medicaid (CMS). Outpatient mental health services include those provided by a private practice mental health professional, outpatient clinic, general medical program or physician, hospital emergency room, outpatient substance abuse treatment program, and other outpatient programs.

[31] Ramesh Ragavan, et al., "Interstate Variation in Psychotropic Medication Use Among Children in the Child Welfare System," *Child Maltreatment*, vol. 15, no. 2, pp. 121-131.

[32] For purposes of Medicaid eligibility "foster care" status extends to some (but not all) children in foster care, most children who are adopted from foster care, and certain children who have aged out of foster care. For further information, "Limitations on Understanding Medicaid Spending for Foster Care Children," in CRS Report R42378, *Child Welfare: Health Care Needs of Children in Foster Care and Related Federal Issues*, by Emilie Stoltzfus et al.

[33] David Rubin et al., "Interstate Variation in Trends of Psychotropic Medication Use Among Medicaid-enrolled Children in Foster Care." This included 47 states and the District of Columbia. See also Julie M. Zito et al., "Psychotropic Medication Patterns Among Youth in Foster Care," *Pediatrics,* vol. 121, no. 1 (July 2008), pp. e157- e163 (hereinafter Julie M. Zito et al., "Psychotropic Medication Patterns Among Youth in Foster Care"); and GAO, *Foster Children: HS Guidance Could Help States Improve Oversight of Psychotropic Prescriptions.*

[34] Congress authorized and funded this longitudinal research in Section 429 of the Social Security Act. NSCAW I, which included five waves of data collection, was conducted between 1999 and 2007. NSCAW II, which included three waves of data collection, was conducted between 2008 and 2012. Congress last provided NSCAW funding for FY2011.

[35] NSCAW II data in this report are based on four sources (1) Heather Ringeisen et al., *NSCAW II Baseline Report: Children's Services* (for data based on four to six months after the investigation); (2) Cecilia Casanueva et al., *NSCAW II Wave 2 Report: Children's Services,* Exhibit 14, Final Report, RTI International for HHS, ACF, Office of Planning, Research and Evaluation, July 2012 (for data based on 18 months after the investigation); (3) correspondence with the U.S. Department of Health and Human Services, Administration for Children and Families, Office of Planning Research and Evaluation (OPRE), January 2014 (for data based on 4 to 6 months, 18 months, and 36 months after the investigation); and (4) Cecilia Casanueva et al., *NSCAW II Wave 3 Report: Wave 3 Tables*, Final Report, RTI International for HHS, ACF, Office of Planning, Research and Evaluation, June 2014 (hereinafter Cecilia Casanueva et al., *NSCAW II Wave 3 Report: Wave 3 Tables*).

[36] Some studies also show a higher rate of psychotropic use among males, compared to females. For example, the NSCAW II data indicate that a far greater percentage of males who had contact with child welfare services (including those who are not removed from the home and placed in foster care) were prescribed psychotropics (14.9% for males versus 8.5% for females) approximately 18 months following the investigation for abuse and neglect. Cecilia Casanueva et al., *NSCAW II Wave 2 Report: Children's Services*, p. 40. Similarly, data from NSCAW I showed somewhat similar results for males in foster care (19.6% versus 7.7%). Ramesh Raghavan et al., "Psychotropic Medication Use in a National Probability Sample of Children in the Child Welfare System," *Journal of Child and Adolescent Psychopharmacology, vol. 15, no. 1*, p. 97.

[37] Based on correspondence with HHS, ACF, OPRE, January 2014.

[38] Heather Ringeisen et al., *NSCAW II Baseline Report: Children's Services*, p. 45.

[39] Cecilia Casanueva et al., *NSCAW II Wave 2 Report: Children's Services*, p. 40; and HHS, ACF, ACYF, *AFCARS Report No. 21*, July 2012. The NSCAW survey data include children in foster care at 18 or 36 months after the initial investigation that brought them to the attention of the child welfare agency. The median time that children remain in foster care is approximately 13 months, and the average stay is 22 months.

[40] Cecilia Casanueva et al., *NSCAW II Wave 3 Report: Wave 3 Tables.*

[41] Cecilia Casanueva et al., *NSCAW II Wave 2 Report: Children's Services.*

[42] Cecilia Casanueva et al., *NSCAW II Wave 3 Report: Wave 3 Tables.*

[43] HHS, ACF, ACYF, CB, "Oversight of Psychotropic Medication for Children in Foster Care; Title IV-B Health Care Oversight & Coordination Plan," April 11, 2012. (Hereinafter HHS, ACF, ACYF, CB, "Oversight of Psychotropic Medication for Children in Foster Care; Title IV-B Health Care Oversight & Coordination Plan.")

[44] David Rubin et al., "Interstate Variation in Trends of Psychotropic Medication Use Among Medicaid-enrolled Children in Foster Care."

[45] Leyla F. Stambaugh et al., *Psychotropic Medication Use by Children in Child Welfare*, p. 4.

[46] Susan dosReis et al., "Antipsychotic Treatment Among Youth in Foster Care," *Pediatrics,* vol. 128, no. 6 (December 2011). (Hereinafter Susan dosReis et al., "Antipsychotic Treatment Among Youth in Foster Care.")

[47] Cecilia Casanueva et al., *NSCAW II Wave 2 Report: Children's Services,* Exhibit 14.

[48] GAO, *Foster Children: HHS Guidance Could Help States Improve Oversight of Psychotropic Prescriptions,* p. 15.

[49] Institute of Medicine of the National Academies, Committee on Crossing the Quality Chasm: Adaptation to Mental Health and Addictive Disorders, *Improving the Quality of Health Care for Mental and Substance-Use Conditions: Quality Chasm Series,* 2006; and Myrna M. Weissman et al., "National Survey of Psychotherapy Training in Psychiatry, Psychology, and Social Work," *Archives of General Psychiatry,* vol. 63 (2006).

[50] The Food and Drug Administration (FDA) approves a drug for sale based on evidence of safety and effectiveness in its intended use, manufacturing requirements, and labeling. Despite the indications for use in the approved labeling, a licensed physician may—except in highly regulated circumstances—prescribe the approved drug without restriction. Prescription to an individual whose demographic or medical characteristics differ from those indicated in a drug's FDA-approved labeling is called off-label use and is accepted medical practice. Off-label use presents an evaluation problem to FDA safety reviewers. Using drugs in new ways for which researchers have not yet demonstrated safety and effectiveness can create problems that premarket studies did not address. Manufacturers rarely design studies to establish the safety and effectiveness of their drugs in off-label uses, and individuals and groups wanting to conduct such studies face difficulties finding funding. FDA's role in making sure a drug is safe and effective continues after the drug is approved and it appears on the market. FDA oversees surveillance, studies, labeling changes, and information dissemination, among other tasks, as long as the drug is sold. For further information, see CRS Report R41983, *How FDA Approves Drugs and Regulates Their Safety and Effectiveness,* by Susan Thaul.

[51] GAO, *Children's Mental Health,* GAO-13-15, December 2012, http://www.gao.gov/products/gao-13-15, pp. 10-11.

[52] Mark Olfson et al., "National Trends in the Mental Health Care of Children, Adolescents, and Adults by Office-Based Physicians."

[53] HHS, Agency for Healthcare Research and Quality, Effective Health Care Program, *First- and Second-Generation Antipsychotics for Children and Young Adults,* Executive Summary, Comparative Effectiveness Review No. 39, February 12, 2012, http://www.effectivehealth care.ahrq.gov/ehc/products/147/835/CER39_Antipsychotics-ChildrenYoung-Adults_ 20120221.pdf.

[54] Leyla F. Stambaugh et al., *Psychotropic Medication Use by Children in Child Welfare.*

[55] JoAnne Solchany, "Psychotropic Medication and Children in Foster Care: Tips for Advocates and Judges," *Child Law Practice,* vol. 31, no. 2 (February 2010), pp. 17, 22-27; HHS, ACF, ACYF, CB, "Promoting Social and Emotional Well-Being for Children and Youth Receiving Child Welfare Services," April 2012.

[56] Barbara J. Burns, Kimberly Hoagwood, and Patricia J. Mrazek, "Effective Treatment for Mental Disorders in Children and Adolescents," vol. 2, no. 4 (1999), pp. 212-213, 232-233.

[57] GAO, *Foster Children: HHS Guidance Could Help States Improve Oversight of Psychotropic Prescriptions.*

[58] U.S Congress, House Ways and Means Subcommittee on Human Resources, *Protection for Foster Children Enrolled in Clinical Trials,* May 18, 2005, 109th Cong., 1st Sess.

[59] Section 6(c) of P.L. 109-288, which added this requirement to Section 422(b)(14) of the Social Security Act.

[60] This subcommittee was previously, and is now, known as the Human Resources subcommittee.

[61] U.S. Congress, House Ways and Means Subcommittee on Income Security and Family Support, *Health Care of Children in Foster Care*, July 19, 2002, 110th Cong., 1st Sess. and *Prescription Psychotropic Drug Use Among Children in Foster Care*, May 8, 2008, 110th Cong., 2nd Sess.

[62] U.S. Congress, Senate Committee on Homeland Security and Governmental Affairs, Subcommittee on Federal Financial Management, Government Information, Federal Services, and International Security, *The Cost of Medicating America's Foster Children*, 112th Cong., 1st sess., December 2011, S. Hrg. 112–448.

[63] GAO, *Foster Children: HHS Guidance Could Help States Improve Oversight of Psychotropic Prescriptions*, GAO-12-270T, December 1, 2011, http://www.gao.gov/products/GAO-12-270T.

[64] American Academy of Child and Adolescent Psychiatry, *AACAP Position Statement on Oversight of Psychotropic Medication Use for Children in State Custody: A Best Principles Guideline*, no date, http://www.aacap.org/ App_Themes/AACAP/docs/member_resources/ practice_information/foster_care/ FosterCare_BestPrinciples_FINAL.pdf. The AACAP guidelines are targeted for children in care and other settings. These guidelines focus on screening and monitoring; continuity of care, effective case management, and longitudinal treatment planning; access to effective psychosocial, psychotherapeutic, and behavioral treatments, and when indicated, pharmacotherapy; consent by the authorized person or agency and assent from the youth; and effective medication management that identifies symptoms, monitors response to treatment, and screens for adverse effects.

[65] These states are Florida, Maryland, Massachusetts, Michigan, Oregon, and Texas.

[66] U.S. Congress, House Committee on Ways and Means, Subcommittee on Human Resources, *Caring for Our Kids: Are We Overmedicating Children in Foster Care?*, 113th Cong., 2nd sess., May 22, 2014.

[67] HHS, *Fiscal Year 2016 Budget: Strengthening Health and Opportunity for All Americans*, February 2015, p. 103. The Administration had the same proposal in the FY2015 budget.

[68] Under the FY2015 proposal, incentive payments would have been paid annually out of the Medicaid program (Title XIX of the Social Security Act) over the five-year period. According to HHS, the incentive payments may be modeled on performance bonuses authorized under the Children's Health Insurance Program Reauthorization Act (CHIPRA). The proposed incentive payments would not have affected how payments are made to Medicaid providers. Those providers would continue to be reimbursed for Medicaid services through normal Medicaid reimbursement procedures. Based on CRS correspondence with U.S. Department of Health and Human Services, Office of the Assistant Secretary for Financial Resources, March 19, 2014.

[69] According to the proposed FY2015 budget, the demonstration sought to serve at least 400,000 children in foster care over the five-year period. States would not have been able to supplant other funds used by the state to carry out the Medicaid state plan, or activities under Titles IV-B or IV-E of the Social Security Act. HHS has explained that the Secretary would have been required to evaluate the demonstration to assess the changes put in place by states; determine whether children in care receive a more appropriate mix of services; and determine whether children's social and emotional functioning is improved. The evaluation would have included a process evaluation, an outcome evaluation, and a cost analysis.

Based on CRS correspondence with U.S. Department of Health and Human Services, Office of the Assistant Secretary for Financial Resources, March 19, 2014.

[70] Leyla F. Stambaugh et al., *Psychotropic Medication Use by Children in Child Welfare.*

[71] HHS, Joint HHS Letter from George Sheldon, Acting Assistant Secretary, ACF; Donald Berwick, Administrator, CMS; and Pamela Hyde, Administrator, SAMHSA to "State Director," November 23, 2011, http://www.childwelfare.gov/systemwide/mentalhealth/effectiveness/jointlettermeds.pdf.

[72] HHS, *Use of Psychotropics Among Children in Foster Care*, webinar series, January and February 2012, http://gucchdtacenter.georgetown.edu/child_welfare-Past.html. The first two parts of the series focused on providing current data and research on the use of psychotropic medications, including data on the age of children using the medications, the types of foster care placements, and polypharmacy. They also included a presentation solely focused on child trauma and its role in treatment approach and prescription of medications. The third webinar presentation discussed the findings of a study by Tufts University on state oversight and how two states, Illinois and Texas, are overseeing psychotropic medication use by children in foster care.

[73] HHS, ACF, ACYF, *Getting Practical: Developing Your State Plan for Psychotropic Medication Management*, webinar series, March through June 2012, http://gucchdtacenter.georgetown.edu/child_welfare.html.

[74] HHS, ACF, CMS, SAMHSA, *Because Minds Matter: Collaborating to Strengthen Management of Psychotropic Medications for Children and Youth in Foster Care*, "Purpose of the Meeting," https://www.childwelfare.gov/systemwide/mentalhealth/effectiveness/mindsmatter.pdf.

[75] HHS, ACF, CMS, SAMHSA, *Because Minds Matter: Collaborating to Strengthen Management of Psychotropic Medications for Children and Youth in Foster Care*, "State Team Handouts," http://www.pal-tech.com/web/ psychotropic/.

[76] HHS, ACF, CMS, SAMHSA, *Because Minds Matter: Collaborating to Strengthen Management of Psychotropic Medications for Children and Youth in Foster Care*, "Plenary PowerPoints and Handouts" and "Workshop PowerPoints and Handouts," http://www.pal-tech.com/web/psychotropic/.

[77] HHS, ACF, ACYF, CB, "Initiative to Improve Access to Needs-Driven, Evidence-Based/Evidence-informed Mental and Behavioral Health Services in Child Welfare," Application HHS-2012-ACF-ACYF-CO-0279, http://www.acf.hhs.gov/grants/open/foa/files/HHS-2012-ACF-ACYF-CO-0279_0.pdf. These funds were awarded under the Adoption Opportunities program. For further information about the grantees, see http://www.acf.hhs.gov/ programs/cb/resource/discretionary-grant-awards-2012.

[78] HHS, ACF, ACYF, CB, "Promoting Well-Being and Adoption After Trauma," Application HHS-2012-ACF-ACYFCO-0637, http://www.acf.hhs.gov/grants/open/foa/view/HHS-2013-ACF-ACYF-CO-0637. These funds were awarded under the Adoption Opportunities program. For further information about the grantees, see http://www.acf.hhs.gov/programs/cb/resource/discretionary-grant-awards-2013.

[79] For example, the American Academy of Child and Adolescent Psychiatry (AACAP), which represents professionals that work in the field of child psychopharmacology, developed basic principles on the psychiatric and pharmacologic treatment of children in care. See American Academy of Child and Adolescent Psychiatry, *AACAP Position Statement on Oversight of Psychotropic Medication Use for Children in State Custody: A Best Principles Guideline*, no date, http://www.aacap.org/App_Themes/AACAP/docs/member_resources/practice_information/foster_care/ FosterCare_BestPrinciples_FINAL.pdf. In addition, the

Reach Institute convened an expert panel to develop best practices for addressing the mental health needs of children involved in child welfare. See Lisa Hunter Romanelli et al., "Best Practices for Mental Health in Child Welfare: Screening, Assessment, and Treatment Guidelines," *Child Welfare*, vol. 88, no. 1 (2009).

[80] HHS, ACF, ACYF, CB, "Oversight of Psychotropic Medication for Children in Foster Care; Title IV-B Health Care Oversight & Coordination

[81] HHS, ACF, ACYF, CB, "Promoting Social and Emotional Well-Being for Children and Youth Receiving Child Welfare Services," Information Memorandum ACYF-CB-IM-12-04, April 17, 2012, http://www.acf.hhs.gov/sites/ default/files/cb/im1204.pdf. (Hereinafter HHS, ACF, ACYF, CB, "Promoting Social and Emotional Well-Being for Children and Youth Receiving Child Welfare Services.")

[82] HHS, CMS, Center for Medicaid and CHIP Services, Informational Bulletin, "Collaborative Efforts and Technical Assistance Resources to Strengthen the Management of Psychotropic Medications for Vulnerable Populations," August 24, 2012, http://medicaid.gov/Federal-Policy-Guidance/Downloads/CIB-08-24-12.pdf.

[83] HHS, ACF, CMS, SAMHSA, "Dear State Director."

[84] Michael W. Naylor, Christine V. Davidson, and D. Jean Ortega-Piron, et al., "Psychotropic Medication Management for Youth in State Care: Consent, Oversight, and Policy Considerations," *Child Welfare*, vol. 86, no. 5 (September/October 2007), pp. 175-192.

[85] Thomas J. Mackie, "Psychotropic Medication Oversight for Youth in Foster Care: A National Perspective on State Child Welfare Policy and Practice Guidelines," *Children and Youth Services Review*, vol. 33., no. 11 (2011) and Laurel K. Leslie et al., *Multi-State Study on Psychotropic Medication Oversight in Foster Care*, Tufts University, Tufts Clinical and Translational Science Institute, September 2010, http://160.109.101.132/icrhps/prodserv/ docs/Executive_Report_09-07-10_348.pdf.

[86] Kathleen Noonan and Dorothy Miller, "Fostering Transparency: A Preliminary Review of "Policy" Governing Psychotropic Medications in Foster Care," *Hastings Law Journal*, vol. 65 (August 2014).

[87] Section 422(a)(15) of the Social Security Act.

[88] Section 475(1)(C) of the Social Security Act.

[89] Section 475(5)(D) of the Social Security Act.

[90] States must develop a five-year Child and Family Services Plan (CFSP) to describe how they intend to provide child welfare-related child and family services, including meeting requirements of child welfare services programs. In addition to program funding for the Child Welfare Services Program, submission of this report is required for states to receive federal formula funding under the Promoting Safe and Stable Families Program (Title IV-B, Subpart 2 of the Social Security Act), Title I of the Child Abuse Prevention and Treatment Act (CAPTA), and the Chafee Foster Care Independence Program, including Education and Training Vouchers. The most recent five-year plan was developed in 2009 to cover FY2010-FY2014. Additionally, in each year other than the year in which the initial CFSP is submitted, the state must submit an Annual Progress and Services Report (APSR) to discuss how the state is accomplishing the goals and objectives of the CFSP and include other assurances related to federal funding for child welfare-related services. Federal regulations at 45 CFR 1357 apply to the CFSP. The CFSP process began in 1994. Since this time, HHS has issued annual Program Instructions (PI) regarding how to meet the CFSP and annual update requirements.

[91] For the report submitted in 2013, states were asked to provide information on these same protocols and to inform HHS whether they have been updated in light of the "Because

Minds Matter" summit hosted by HHS in August 2012. For the final report submitted for the FY2010 through FY2014 period, and the CFSP for FY2015 through FY2019, HHS requested information about the oversight of prescription medicines, including protocols for the appropriate use and monitoring of psychotropic medications.

[92] Thirty-seven states have APSRs with final dates that are between July and November 2012.

[93] Polypharmacy is the practice of prescribing multiple drugs to be taken concurrently to treat one or more health problems. *Mosby's Dictionary of Medicine, Nursing, & Health Professions*, "polypharmacy," http://www.credoreference.com/entry/ehsmosbymed/polypharmacy; *Dictionary of Medical Terms*, "polypharmacy," http://www.credoreference.com/entry/acbmedterm/polypharmacy.

[94] HHS, SAMHSA, "Health Homes," http://beta.samhsa.gov/health-reform/health-care-integration/health-homes; HHS, SAMHSA, "What Is a Health Home?" SAMHSA Blog, December 4, 2010, http://blog.samhsa.gov/2010/12/04/what-isa-health-home/; HHS, SAMHSA, "Health Homes: A Strategy to Improve Care," *SAMHSA News*, vol. 12, no. 2 (Spring 2013), http://www.samhsa.gov/samhsaNewsLetter/Volume_21_Number_2/improve_care.aspx; HHS, CMS, "Health Homes," Medicaid.gov, http://www.medicaid.gov/Medicaid-CHIP-Program-Information/By-Topics/Long-TermServices-and-Support/Integrating-Care/Health-Homes/Health-Homes.html.

[95] For a list of these State Plan Amendments, see http://www.medicaid.gov/State-Resource-Center/Medicaid-StateTechnical-Assistance/Health-Homes-Technical-Assistance/Approved-Health-Home-State-Plan-Amendments.html.

[96] HHS, ACF, ACYF, CB, "Oversight of Psychotropic Medication for Children in Foster Care; Title IV-B Health Care Oversight & Coordination.

[97] See for example, information about a statewide medical home model in Illinois: Paula Kienberger Jaudes et al., "Expanding medical home model works for children in foster care," *Child Welfare*, vol. 91, no. 1 (2012), pp. 9-33.

[98] HHS, ACF, ACYF, CB, Program Instruction ACYF-CB-PI-12-05, April 11, 2012, p. 12, available at http://www.acf.hhs.gov/sites/default/files/cb/pi1205.pdf.

[99] HHS, ACF, ACYF, CB, Information Memorandum ACYF-CB-IM-12-03, April 11, 2012, p. 16, http://www.acf.hhs.gov/sites/default/files/cb/im1203.pdf.

[100] For further information, see CRS Report R40161, *The Health Information Technology for Economic and Clinical Health (HITECH) Act*, by C. Stephen Redhead.

[101] HHS, ACF, CMS, SAMHSA, "Dear State Director," July 2013.

[102] HHS, OIG, "Most Medicaid Children in Nine States Are Not Receiving All Required Preventive Screening Services," May 2010 (OEI-05-08-00520). The report cited a need for improved documentation of certain screenings as well as better provider knowledge of what a screening entails (among other things) as ways to improve services. In December 2010, CMS convened a National EPSDT Improvement Workgroup to help identify areas for improvement of EPSDT and to work at the federal level and with states to improve both children's access to EPSDT services and the quality of the data reporting on receipt of those services. See http://www.medicaid.gov/Medicaid-CHIP-ProgramInformation/By-Topics/Benefits/Early-Periodic-Screening-Diagnosis-and-Treatment.html.

[103] GAO, *Children's Mental Health: Concerns Remain about Appropriate Services for Children in Medicaid and Foster Care*, GAO-13-15, December 2015, pp. 23-24. HHS, CMS, Center for Medicaid and CHIP Services, "Prevention and Early Identification of Mental Health and Substance Use Conditions," Informational Bulletin, March 27, 2013, http://www.medicaid.gov/federal-policy-guidance/downloads/CIB-03-27-2013.pdf.

[104] In guidance to state child welfare agencies, HHS has emphasized foster children's eligibility for screening and other services under the EPSDT program. See U.S. Department of Health and Human Services, Administration for Children and Families, Administration for Children, Youth and Families, Children's Bureau, "Promoting Social and Emotional Well-Being for Children and Youth Receiving Child Welfare Services."

[105] HHS, CMS, Center for Medicaid and CHIP Services, "Drug Utilization Review," http://www.medicaid.gov/Medicaid-CHIP-Program-Information/By-Topics/Benefits/Prescription-Drugs/Drug-Utilization-Review.html; Informational Bulletin, August 24, 2012, http://www.medicaid.gov/Federal-Policy-Guidance/downloads/CIB-08-24- 12.pdf.

[106] Bryan Samuels, [former] Commissioner, HHS, ACF, ACYF, "Strengthening Psychotropic Medication Management: Another Step in Improving Well-Being of Children in Foster Care." *Because Minds Matter: Collaborating to Strengthen Management of Psychotropic Medications for Children and Youth in Foster Care.*

[107] American Academy of Child & Adolescent Psychiatry, "Youth Voice Tip Sheet, Communication Between Child and Adolescent Psychiatrist & Youth: 10 Tips to Improve the Conversation," January 2012, http://www.aacap.org/ App_Themes/AACAP/docs/youth_resources/misc/Youth_Voice_Tip_Sheet_2012.pdf.

[108] Thirty-seven states have APSRs with final dates that are between July and November 2012.

[109] At least one study refers to a "mental health evaluation" for children in foster care as "screening and/or assessment for emotional and behavioral problems." In Laurel K. Leslie et al., *Multi-State Study on Psychotropic Medication Oversight in Foster Care*, Tufts University, Tufts Clinical and Translational Science Institute, September 2010, http://160.109.101.132/icrhps/prodserv/docs/Executive_Report_09-07-10_348.pdf.

[110] Nearly all children in foster care are eligible for Medicaid, which is a means-tested entitlement program administered by the federal government in partnership with states. Medicaid finances the delivery of primary and acute medical services as well as long-term care. Anne M. Libby et al., "Child Welfare Systems Policies and Practices Affecting Medicaid Health Insurance for Children: A National Study," *Journal of Social Science Research*, vol. 33, no. 2 (2006), p. 33.

[111] Children in foster care are categorically eligible for Medicaid because they qualify for assistance under the Title IV-E foster care program, or via other mandatory or optional pathways that are available under each state's Medicaid plan. Children in care are generally entitled to the same set of "traditional" Medicaid state plan services available to other categorically needy children enrolled in a given state's Medicaid program. Central among these benefits is a provision in the law requiring that children receive all medically necessary services authorized in federal statute through the Early and Periodic Screening, Diagnosis, and Treatment (EPSDT) program. The EPSDT program covers health screenings and services, including assessments of each child's physical development and mental health; laboratory tests (including screening blood lead test); appropriate immunizations; health education; and vision, dental, and hearing services. The screenings and services must be provided at regular intervals that meet "reasonable" medical or dental practice standards.

[112] Committee on Bioethics, "Informed Consent, Parental Permission, and Assent in Pediatric Practice," *Pediatrics,* vol. 95, no. 2 (February 1995), pp. 314-318; *A.D.A.M. Medical Encyclopedia,* "informed consent," http://www.nlm.nih.gov/ medlineplus/ency/patientinstructions/000445.htm; *Oxford Concise Medical Dictionary,* 8th ed., "assent," http://www.oxfordreference.com/view/10.1093/acref/9780199557141.001.0001/acref-9780199557141-e-11145; Laurel K. Leslie et al., *Multi-State Study on Psychotropic Medication Oversight in Foster Care,* Tufts University, Tufts Clinical and Translational

Science Institute, September 2010, http://160.109.101.132/icrhps/prodserv/docs/ Executive_Report_09-07-10_348.pdf.

[113] Polypharmacy is the practice of prescribing multiple drugs to be taken concurrently to treat one or more health problems. *Mosby's Dictionary of Medicine, Nursing, & Health Professions*, "polypharmacy," http://www.credoreference.com/entry/ehsmosbymed/ polypharmacy; *Dictionary of Medical Terms*, "polypharmacy," http://www.credoreference. com/entry/acbmedterm/polypharmacy.

[114] Medicaid.gov, Drug Utilization Review, http://www.medicaid.gov/Medicaid-CHIP-Program- Information/ByTopics/Benefits/Prescription-Drugs/Drug-Utilization-Review.html; Center for Medicaid and CHIP Services, Informational Bulletin, August 24, 2012, http://www.medicaid.gov/Federal-Policy-Guidance/downloads/CIB-08-24- 12.pdf

[115] American Board of Psychiatry and Neurology, Inc., "Frequently Asked Questions," no date, http://www.abpn.com/ faqs.html.

[116] American Board of Medical Specialties, "Board Certification Editorial Background," March 29, 2013, http://www.abms.org/news_and_events/media_newsroom/pdf/abms_editorial background.pdf. This document states that "[t]he amount of time a candidate can declare him/herself as Board Eligible ranges from five to seven years, depending on the Member Board." The American Board of Psychiatry and Neurology has set the time limit at seven years. See "ABMS Member Boards' Board Eligibility Periods and Transition Dates," http://www.abms.org/ News_and_Events/downloads/ABMS_Board_Eligibility_Policy_ by_Board_021313.pdf.

In: Psychotropic Medication …
Editor: Malcolm C. Burgess

ISBN: 978-1-63485-155-8
© 2016 Nova Science Publishers, Inc.

Chapter 2

FOSTER CHILDREN: ADDITIONAL FEDERAL GUIDANCE COULD HELP STATES BETTER PLAN FOR OVERSIGHT OF PSYCHOTROPIC MEDICATIONS ADMINISTERED BY MANAGED-CARE ORGANIZATIONS*

United States Government Accountability Office

ABBREVIATIONS

AACAP	American Academy of Child and Adolescent Psychiatry
ACF	Administration for Children and Families
ADHD	attention deficit hyperactivity disorder
APSR	Annual Progress and Services Report
CANS	Child and Adolescent Needs and Strengths
CHIP	State Children's Health Insurance Program
CMS	Centers for Medicare and Medicaid
EPSDT	Early and Periodic Screening, Diagnostic, and Treatment
FDA	Food and Drug Administration
HHS	Department of Health and Human Services
MCO	managed-care organization

---

* This is an edited, reformatted and augmented version of The United States Government Accountability Office publication, GAO-14-362, dated April 2014.

OIG   Office of Inspector General
PTSD   post-traumatic stress disorder
SAMHSA   Substance Abuse and Mental Health Services Administration

WHY GAO DID THIS STUDY

In December 2011, GAO reported that foster children in selected states were prescribed psychotropic medications at rates higher than nonfoster children in Medicaid in 2008. GAO was asked to further examine instances of foster children being prescribed psychotropic medications.

For the five states included in GAO's 2011 report—Florida, Massachusetts, Michigan, Oregon, and Texas—this report: (1) assesses the extent that documentation supported the usage of psychotropic medication for selected cases; and (2) describes states' policies related to psychotropic medication and assesses HHS actions since GAO's 2011 report.

GAO contracted with two child psychiatrists who conduct mental-health research and work on issues related to foster care, to provide clinical evaluations of 24 cases that GAO selected from the population of foster children prescribed psychotropic drugs in GAO's 2011 report. The case selections were based, in part, on potential health risk indicators, and the findings are not generalizable. GAO obtained medical and child-welfare documentation spanning children's time in foster care, and redacted personally identifiable information prior to experts' review of cases. GAO also analyzed federal guidance and selected states' policies and interviewed federal and state officials.

WHAT GAO RECOMMENDS

GAO recommends that HHS issue guidance to states regarding oversight of psychotropic medications prescribed to children in foster care through MCOs. HHS agreed with GAO's recommendation.

WHAT GAO FOUND

Two experts GAO contracted with reviewed foster and medical records for 24 cases in five selected states and found varying quality in the documentation supporting the use of psychotropic medications for children in foster care. Experts examined documentation related to several categories, such as (1) screening, assessment, and treatment planning; and (2) medication monitoring.

- *Screening, Assessment, and Treatment Planning.* Experts' evaluation of this category included whether medical pediatric exams and evidence-based therapies—which are interventions shown to produce measureable improvements—were provided as needed, according to records. Experts found in 22 of 24 cases that medical pediatric exams were mostly supported by documentation. For example, in one case with mostly supporting documentation, experts found that a child with a history of behavioral and emotional problems had records documenting a medical pediatric exam and thorough psychological assessments, with comprehensive discussions of diagnostic issues and medication rationale. With regard to evidence-based therapies, experts found that 3 of 15 children who may have benefitted from such therapies were mostly provided such services, while 11 of 15 cases were scored as partial in this category, and in 1 of 15 cases there was no documentation that evidence-based therapies were provided.
- *Medication Monitoring.* Experts' evaluation of this category included the appropriateness of medication dosage and the rationale for concurrent use of multiple medications, according to records. Experts found appropriateness of medication dosages was mostly supported by documentation in 13 of 24 cases and partially supported in the other 11 cases. The rationale for concurrent use of multiple medications was mostly supported in 5 of the 20 cases where multiple medications were used, but 14 of 20 cases included documentation that partially supported concurrent use, and 1 case did not include documentation to support concurrent use. For example, experts found for one case that a child was prescribed four psychotropic drugs concurrently, when nonmedication interventions could have been considered. The rationale for the actions taken was partially supported by documentation.

All of the five selected states—two of which pay health care providers directly through fee-for-service, and three of which use or are transitioning to a third-party managed-care organization (MCO) for prescription-drug benefits to some extent—have policies intended to address oversight of psychotropic medications for foster children. According to state officials, all five of the states require medical examinations for children in foster care. Since GAO's 2011 report, the Department of Health and Human Services' (HHS) Administration for Children and Families (ACF) has, among other things, worked with other federal agencies to provide informational webinars and technical guidance for states to improve oversight of psychotropic medications, but this guidance does not address third-party MCOs administering medications. Officials from two of the three states relying on MCOs described limited state planning for MCOs to monitor psychotropic medications. Because there are indications MCO use is increasing, additional HHS guidance that helps states implement oversight strategies within the context of a managed-care environment could help ensure appropriate monitoring of psychotropic medications prescribed to children in foster care.

* * *

April 28, 2014

Congressional Requesters

Children in foster care with mental-health conditions are among the country's most vulnerable populations, and there are concerns about whether they have access to the most appropriate care for their conditions.[1] Early detection and treatment of emotional and behavioral disturbances can improve a child's symptoms and reduce potentially detrimental effects on a child, such as difficulties with relationships, dropping out of school, and involvement with the juvenile justice system. Children with mental-health conditions, such as attention deficit hyperactivity disorder (ADHD) or depression, can be treated with psychosocial therapies (sessions with a provider designed to reduce symptoms and improve functioning); psychotropic medication (medications that affect mood, thought, or behavior); or a combination of both.

Child mental-health advocates, providers, and researchers have expressed concern about the increase in the prescription of psychotropic medications to children, due in part to limited evidence available regarding short- and long-term safety and efficacy for some types of medications, particularly when used in combination. Some state Medicaid and mental-health officials have expressed concern about the relatively high rates of off-label use of antipsychotics, particularly among groups of special concern such as children in foster care.[2]

Several agencies in the Department of Health and Human Services (HHS) have responsibilities related to children's mental health. The Administration for Children and Families (ACF) provides funding for and oversees states' child-welfare programs, which are responsible for monitoring and coordinating mental-health services for children in foster care, among other things. The Centers for Medicare & Medicaid Services (CMS) oversees, and jointly finances with the states, Medicaid and the State Children's Health Insurance Program (CHIP), which provide health coverage for low-income children. State Medicaid programs are required by federal law to provide coverage for certain health services, which may include mental-health services, for children through the Early and Periodic Screening, Diagnostic, and Treatment (EPSDT) benefit. The Substance Abuse and Mental Health Services Administration (SAMHSA) works to increase the quality and availability of mental-health services, such as by awarding grants that support the development of community-based services for children with mental-health conditions, including children in foster care.

Children in foster care who are enrolled in Medicaid may receive services generally through one of two distinct service-delivery and financing systems—managed care or fee-for-service. Under a managed-care model, states contract with a managed-care organization (MCO) and prospectively pay the plans a fixed monthly fee per patient to provide or arrange for most health services, which may include prescription-drug benefits. Plans, in turn, pay providers. In the traditional fee-for-service delivery system, the Medicaid program reimburses providers directly and on a retrospective basis for each service delivered.

In December 2011, we reported that children in foster care in the five states analyzed were prescribed psychotropic medications at higher rates than nonfoster children in Medicaid during 2008.[3] According to research, experts consulted, and certain federal and state officials interviewed as part of our December 2011 report, this could be due in part to foster children's greater exposure to traumatic experiences, and the challenges of coordinating their medical care and records due to frequent changes in placement. Prescriptions to foster children in these states were also more likely to have indicators of potential health risks. According to the experts we consulted for our December 2011 report, no evidence supports the concurrent use of five or more psychotropic medications in adults or children, yet hundreds of both foster and nonfoster children in the five states had such a drug regimen. Similarly, in our December 2011 report, we found thousands of foster and nonfoster children were prescribed doses higher than the maximum levels cited in guidelines developed by the state of Texas, based on Food and Drug Administration (FDA)– approved or medical literature maximum dosages for children and adolescents, which experts said increases the risk of adverse side effects and does not typically increase the efficacy of the medications to any significant extent.[4] We also found that the monitoring programs of these states for psychotropic medications provided to children in foster care varied and fell short of best-principles guidelines published by the American Academy of Child and Adolescent Psychiatry (AACAP).[5] This variation was expected because states set their own guidelines and HHS had not endorsed specific measures for state oversight of psychotropic prescriptions for children in foster care. In our December 2011 report we recommended, and HHS agreed, to consider endorsing guidance for states on best practices for overseeing psychotropic prescriptions for children in foster care. The status of this recommendation is discussed later in this report.

You asked us to continue our review of psychotropic medications provided to children in foster care. This report (1) examines the extent to which the use of psychotropic medications was supported by foster and medical records for selected case studies of children in foster care who were prescribed these medications; and (2) describes selected states' policies or procedures intended to address oversight of psychotropic medications, and assesses what, if any, actions HHS has taken to help states oversee psychotropic medications prescribed to children in foster care since our December 2011 report.

To examine the extent to which the use of psychotropic medications was supported by foster and medical records, we selected a nonrepresentative sample of 28 children in foster care covered by Medicaid in Florida, Massachusetts, Michigan, Oregon, and Texas in 2008.[6] Thus, the results of our case-study analysis are not generalizable to the foster-child population within each of the five states we examined, or to those of other states.

For each state included in our review, we randomly selected four cases; each case represented one of the following four categories:

- children prescribed any psychotropic medication during calendar year 2008 and in foster care as of January 2010;

- children with prescriptions exceeding dosage guidelines developed by the state of Texas, which were based on FDA-approved or medical literature maximum dosages for children and adolescents, during calendar year 2008 and in foster care as of January 2010;
- children prescribed five or more medications concurrently during calendar year 2008 and in foster care as of January 2010; and
- children less than 1 year old prescribed any psychotropic medication during calendar year 2008 and in foster care as of January 2010.

In addition to the 20 cases above, we also nonrandomly selected all children less than 1 year old prescribed an ADHD, antipsychotic, or antidepressant medication during calendar year 2008, totaling 8 infants. These additional 8 cases were selected because, according to experts, it is not standard practice to prescribe psychotropic medications to infants, and these medications carry significant risks when prescribed to young children.

After preliminary analysis, we excluded four selected cases from our review. One case removed was a nonrandomly selected infant case in which the prescription was identified as potential Medicaid fraud and the case was referred to the state Medicaid Office of Inspector General for follow up. Two other nonrandomly selected infant cases were removed due to data-entry errors that indicated children received psychotropic medications, when they had not.[7] The fourth case removed was a randomly selected infant case. In this case, the records provided did not include any mental-health or prescription information for experts to review. State officials confirmed the psychotropic medication prescribed to the infant was for non-mental-health purposes. Thus, 24 cases were included in our final case-file review.

To provide a clinical perspective on our cases, we contracted with two child psychiatrists who are board certified in child and adolescent psychiatry, have conducted clinical research regarding mental illness in children, and who are working on issues related to psychotropic medication use among children in foster care. For additional information on experts and the criteria that informed our selection, see appendix I. To review the cases, the two experts collaborated to develop categories that are applicable to the administration of psychotropic medications, as informed by AACAP guidelines and their clinical experience. The categories include, but are not limited to, the quality of documentation related to psychiatric evaluations, monitoring and efficacy of medications, and changes in medication doses.[8] GAO obtained medical and child-welfare documentation spanning the children's time in foster care, and redacted personally identifiable information prior to experts' review of cases.

For each case, experts reviewed the child's medical and foster care information (such as case-file notes, medical history, and prescriptions) covering the entire period the child was in foster care, and provided an opinion on the categories reviewed, as well as a summary narrative describing the facts and circumstances surrounding the child's use of psychotropic medication.[9] Experts noted any potential issues related to the use of psychotropic medications based on supporting documentation, which was reviewed from a quantitative and qualitative standpoint. The experts' opinions are presented topically using ACF's program instructions regarding (1) screening, assessment, and treatment planning; (2) medication monitoring; and (3) informed and shared decision making as a framework to illustrate case findings.

We provided officials from selected states with copies of the experts' preliminary case reviews to help ensure all available documentation was included for experts' evaluations and to allow state experts, including experts in child and adolescent psychiatry, to review the expert case descriptions. State officials were given an opportunity to provide additional comments or documentation, and we incorporated their comments into this report as appropriate.

To describe the five selected states' policies or procedures intended to provide oversight of psychotropic medications and determine what, if any, actions HHS has taken to help states oversee psychotropic medications prescribed to foster children since December 2011, we reviewed federal statutes, regulations, and state policies related to the prescribing and oversight of psychotropic medications to foster children. We also interviewed officials from ACF, CMS, and SAMHSA, as well as child-welfare and Medicaid officials from selected states, to understand their approach to providing oversight of psychotropic medications. We assessed HHS's efforts, including guidance provided to state Medicaid and child-welfare programs regarding the monitoring of psychotropic medications prescribed to children in foster care, using GAO's *Standards for Internal Control in the Federal Government*.[10] We did not evaluate the extent to which the five selected states' procedures were being implemented effectively.

We conducted this performance audit from January 2012 through April 2014 in accordance with generally accepted government auditing standards. Those standards require that we plan and perform the audit to obtain sufficient, appropriate evidence to provide a reasonable basis for our audit findings and conclusions based on our audit objectives. We believe that the evidence obtained provides a reasonable basis for our findings and conclusions based on our audit objectives.

BACKGROUND

Children enter state foster care when they have been removed from their parents or guardians and placed under the responsibility of a state child-welfare agency. Removal from the home can occur because of reasons such as abuse or neglect. When children are taken into foster care, the state's child-welfare agency becomes responsible for determining where the child should live and providing the child with needed support. The agency may place the foster child in the home of a relative, with unrelated foster parents, or in a group home or residential treatment center, depending on the child's needs. The agency is also responsible for arranging needed services, including mental-health services. Coordinating mental-health care for children in foster care may be difficult for both the medical provider and the caseworker depending on the complexity of the child's needs, and because multiple people are making decisions on the child's behalf. In addition, caseworkers in child-welfare agencies may have large caseloads, making it difficult for them to ensure each child under their authority receives adequate mental-health services.

In 2011, the Child and Family Services Improvement and Innovation Act amended the Social Security Act to require states to identify protocols for monitoring foster children's use of psychotropic medications and to address how emotional trauma associated with children's maltreatment and removal from their homes will be monitored and treated.[11] ACF requires states to address these issues in their required Annual Progress and Services Reports (APSR) and has provided guidance detailing how states are to address protocols for monitoring foster children's use of psychotropic medications as part of the state's APSR.[12] Among other things, state monitoring protocols are to address

- screening, assessment, and treatment planning to identify children's mental-health and trauma-treatment needs, including a psychiatric evaluation, as necessary, to identify needs for psychotropic medications;
- effective medication monitoring at both the client and agency level; and

- informed and shared decision making and methods for ongoing communication between the prescriber, the child, caregivers, other health care providers, the child-welfare worker, and other key stakeholders.

According to ACF, child-welfare systems that choose to pursue comprehensive and integrated approaches to screening, assessing, and addressing children's behavioral and mental-health needs—including the effects of childhood traumatic experiences—are more likely to increase children's sense of safety and provide them with effective care. In particular, ACF, CMS, and SAMHSA noted the role of evidence-based practices—interventions shown to produce measureable improvements or promising results—in decreasing emotional or behavioral symptoms. In addition, according to ACF, psychotropic medication use with young children, including infants, is of special concern since this population may be especially vulnerable to adverse effects, necessitating careful management and oversight.

As we reported in December 2011, oversight procedures such as prescription monitoring help states to identify and review potentially risky prescribing practices in the foster-care population.[13] Monitoring for appropriate dosage can be beneficial as it is important for any medication or combination of medications prescribed to use appropriate dosages to maximize the likelihood of effectiveness while also minimizing the chance of potential adverse effects. Monitoring for concurrent use of multiple psychotropic medications can be beneficial because, according to ACF, there is little evidence of the effectiveness of using multiple psychotropic medications at the same time and no research to support the use of five or more psychotropic medications.

According to AACAP, treatment planning should include discussions by key stakeholders, such as prescribers and caregivers, about the assessment of target symptoms, behaviors, function, and potential benefits and adverse effects of treatment options. As we reported in December 2011, informed consent helps ensure that caregivers are fully aware of the risks and benefits associated with the decision to medicate with psychotropic medications and to accurately assess and monitor the foster child's reaction to the medications.[14]

CASE STUDIES VARIED IN QUALITY OF DOCUMENTATION SUPPORTING THE USE OF PSYCHOTROPIC MEDICATIONS

Expert reviews of 24 foster children's foster and medical files in five selected states found that the quality of documentation supporting the prescription of psychotropic medication usage varied with respect to (1) screening, assessment, and treatment planning; (2) medication monitoring; and (3) informed and shared decision making.

Quality of Documentation to Support Sufficient Screening, Assessment, and Treatment Planning Varied among Selected Cases

For each of our 24 cases, experts evaluated the foster and medical records across six categories they developed collaboratively that relate to screening, assessment, and treatment planning and provided their professional opinion for the case. Examples of screening, assessment, and treatment planning categories reviewed include the extent to which medical examinations, psychiatric evaluations, and evidence-based therapies were provided, and whether the impact of trauma was addressed by treatment.[15] As shown in table 1, experts found that the quality of screening, assessment, and treatment planning varied among selected cases according to documentation reviewed. To see how experts scored all six categories, see appendix II.

Experts found that medical pediatric examinations were mostly supported by documentation for 22 of 24 cases. Experts found in 2 of 24 cases the medical pediatric examinations were partially supported, such as when the medical pediatric exams were mentioned in the documentation, but not actually included in the records, preventing experts from evaluating what the examinations consisted of, and whether monitoring for psychotropic agents, such as assessing height, weight, or laboratory functions, was conducted. In one example, whereby experts scored the medical pediatric exam category as mostly supported in documentation, a child with a history of behavioral and emotional problems—including aggression and hyperactivity—was prescribed multiple ADHD medications. In this case, experts noted the child's records had thorough psychological and pediatric assessments, with comprehensive discussions of diagnostic issues and medication rationale as well as good case-management summaries.

Table 1. Quality of Documentation Support Related to Screening, Assessment, and Treatment Planning

Category	Mostly supported in foster file or medical records	Partially supported in foster file or medical records	Not supported in foster file or medical records	Not applicable	Total applicablecases
Medical pediatric examination	22	2	0	0	24
Psychiatric evaluations	12	3	2	7	17
Evidence-based therapies provided	3	11	1	9	15
Impact of trauma addressed by treatment	3	8	3	10	14

Source: Expert reviewers.

Notes: The data are from expert reviews of foster file and medical records for 24 selected cases. Experts reviewed each of the categories from a quantitative and qualitative standpoint and provided their consensus evaluation based on documentation reviewed. The case selections include children prescribed a psychotropic drug as of 2008 and in foster care as of 2010 (nonrandomly selected infants did not have the 2010 restriction); however, the experts reviewed foster and medical information from the entire time the child was in foster care, which included the most-recent records available. Experts used the categorization "mostly supported in foster file or medical records" for instances where the documentation reviewed met both quantitative and qualitative measures as deemed appropriate by experts. Experts used the categorization "partially supported in foster file or medical records" for instances where the documentation included some information for the assessed category, but the documentation was either quantitatively or qualitatively, or both, lacking in some regard, according to experts. Experts used the categorization "not supported in foster file or medical records" for instances where there was no documentation for the assessed category, or the information provided was deemed substantively lacking by experts.

Medical Pediatric Examinations

Experts found that psychiatric evaluations were mostly documented for 12 of 17 applicable cases. Experts found 3 of 17 cases had partial documentation to support that the child had received a full psychiatric supported by documentation for 22 of 24 cases. Experts found in 2 of 24 cases the medical pediatric examinations were partially supported, such as when the medical pediatric exams were mentioned in the documentation, but not actually included in the records, preventing experts from evaluating what the examinations consisted of, and whether monitoring for psychotropic agents, such as assessing height, weight, or laboratory functions, was conducted. In one example, whereby experts scored the medical pediatric exam category as mostly supported in documentation, a child with a history of behavioral and emotional problems—including aggression and hyperactivity—was prescribed multiple ADHD medications. In this case, experts noted the child's records had thorough psychological and pediatric assessments, with comprehensive discussions of diagnostic issues and medication rationale as well as good case-management summaries.

Psychiatric Evaluations

Experts found that psychiatric evaluations were mostly documented for 12 of 17 applicable cases. Experts found 3 of 17 cases had partial documentation to support that the child had received a full psychiatric evaluation and 2 of 17 cases had no evidence that a psychiatric evaluation took place. For example, in 1 case with mostly supporting documentation, experts found that a child with a history of disruptive behavior, poor impulse control, anger outbursts, and sexual acting-out behaviors, among other things, received comprehensive psychosocial, psychosexual, and neuropsychological evaluations. Moreover, experts noted the child received special educational services and intensive therapeutic services, and visited a psychiatrist monthly for several months, then was referred back to the pediatrician with scheduled psychiatric check-ins as appropriate.

Evidence-Based Therapies

Experts found that documentation reviewed supported that evidence-based therapies were mostly provided in 3 of 15 applicable cases where the child may have benefited from such treatment. However, in 11 of 15 cases, the experts scored the category as partial, such as for instances when some psychosocial or evidence-based therapies were documented as provided, but other evidence-based therapies that may have been more applicable or beneficial to the child were not provided, based on documents reviewed. In 1 of 15 cases, there was no documentation that evidence-based therapies were provided. In one case, experts found that a child initially placed in foster care as a toddler with over 10 foster-care placements—including group care from 14 to 16 years of age—had experienced early neglect, exposure to domestic violence, and physical abuse, and suffered from severe mood swings and explosive outbursts of anger. According to experts, a larger focus on evidence-based treatments such as trauma-focused cognitive behavioral therapy would have likely benefitted the child, but there was no documentation showing this occurred. However, according to the experts' evaluation of the documentation, the child's psychiatric diagnoses and medication regimens were stable over time, and treatment response, level of treatment intensity, and level of psychosocial functioning were all evaluated appropriately.

In another example, experts found that a child removed from the home at age 13 after being physically assaulted by his mother and witnessing domestic violence received supportive psychotherapy and counseling, but there was no documentation of evidence-based psychotherapies, such as trauma-focused cognitive behavioral therapy. In addition, the forms used to document the therapy each represented 1 month of treatment with progress notes from each of the four weekly sessions. However, the report of the sessions, and often the entire content of the month's psychotherapeutic work, was duplicated for months at a time. One week's psychotherapy content was duplicated for over 1 year, raising questions about what services were actually provided.

Impact of Trauma Addressed by Treatment

Experts found the documentation reviewed supported that the impact of trauma was mostly addressed by treatment for 3 of 14 applicable cases. However, for 8 of 14 cases, the impact of trauma was partially addressed by the treatment provided to children who had suffered from traumatic events, and in 3 cases there was no evidence that the trauma was addressed, according to documentation reviewed. For example, experts found in one case with no supporting documentation, that a child was placed in foster care at 5 years of age for neglect and physical abuse and diagnosed with a variety of different psychiatric conditions, including bipolar disorder, post-traumatic stress disorder (PTSD), schizotypal[16] personality disorder, paranoia, and possible psychosis. According to experts, psychosis and personality disorders are typically considered adult conditions, and are usually not diagnosed in younger children. In this case, the child was treated with variable combinations of ADHD medications, antidepressants, anticonvulsants, and antipsychotics. While hospitalized at age 9 years, the child received an ADHD and antipsychotic medication at dosages that exceeded dosage guidelines based on FDA-approved or medical literature maximum dosages for this age group, and the medications were elevated to these high dosages over a 1 week period. During this time, the child's brother died, yet this was not addressed or acknowledged during the psychiatric hospitalization, according to documentation.[17]

In another example, experts found that a child placed in foster care at 9 years of age due to neglect, physical abuse, and exposure to social chaos and domestic violence received treatment that partially addressed the impact of trauma on the child, according to documentation reviewed. In this case the child reported additional trauma, saying his mother's boyfriend forced him to engage in sexual behavior with his sister. The child's grandmother, who had been his caretaker, also died when he was 13 years old. Experts noted the history of trauma was acknowledged, but an evidence-based intervention was not provided to address the trauma, according to documents reviewed.

Quality of Documentation Supporting Medication Monitoring Varied among Selected Cases

For each case, experts reviewed and provided their opinions across seven categories related to medication monitoring, including the extent to which prescriptions were appropriately monitored by medical providers, appropriate dosages were used, and concurrent use of multiple medications was justified based on documentation reviewed.[18] As shown in table 2, experts found that the quality of prescription monitoring by medical providers, and justification for dosage and concurrent use of multiple medications, varied among selected cases, based on documentation reviewed. See appendix II for a full listing of all categories experts reviewed related to medication monitoring.

Table 2. Quality of Documentation Support Related to Medication Monitoring

Category	Mostly supported in foster file or medical records	Partially supported in foster file or medical records	Not supported in foster file or medical records	Not applicable	Total applicablecases
Prescriptions appropriately monitored	13	9	2	0	24
Appropriate dosages used	13	11	0	0	24
Concurrent use of multiple medications justified	5	14	1	4	20

Source: Expert reviewers.

Notes: The data are from expert reviews of foster file and medical records for 24 selected cases. Experts reviewed each of the categories from a quantitative and qualitative standpoint and provided their consensus evaluation based on documentation reviewed. The case selections include children prescribed a psychotropic drug as of 2008 and in foster care as of 2010 (nonrandomly selected infants did not have the 2010 restriction); however, the experts reviewed foster and medical information from the entire time the child was in foster care, which included the most-recent records available. Experts used the categorization "mostly supported in foster file or medical records" for instances where the documentation reviewed met both quantitative and qualitative measures as deemed appropriate by experts. Experts used the categorization "partially supported in foster file or medical records" for instances where the documentation included some information for the assessed category, but the documentation was either quantitatively or qualitatively, or both, lacking in some regard, according to experts. Experts used the categorization "not supported in foster file or medical records" for instances where there was no documentation for the assessed category, or the information provided was deemed substantively lacking by experts.

Prescriptions Appropriately Monitored

Experts found in 13 of 24 cases that prescriptions were mostly monitored by medical providers based on documentation reviewed. However, in 9 of 24 cases the prescriptions were partially monitored, and in 2 other cases there was no evidence that prescriptions were monitored by medical providers, according to documentation reviewed. For example, experts found in one case with partially supporting documentation that the monitoring of height, weight, vital signs, and metabolic effects of antipsychotic medications was lacking and that the records did not provide an adequate overview of medication risks and concerns regarding concurrent use of multiple psychotropic medications. According to the experts, these factors are important for medical providers to monitor in order to better assess the potential adverse effects of the medication and adjust as necessary to improve patient outcomes. In this case, the child entered foster care at 3 years of age and was noted to be aggressive, oppositional, not sleeping well, and hyperactive. Experts noted some of the antipsychotic prescriptions (quetiapine and olanzapine) were given "as needed" rather than scheduled, which, according to experts, is not considered a good medical practice in a traditional foster-care setting. Experts described the medication management as extremely aggressive, with complicated regimens and dosages at or above the standard recommendations. Furthermore, documentation that the medications were effective was lacking.

Appropriate Dosages Used

For 13 of the 24 cases, experts found that the dosages were mostly supported for the children's medications based on documentation reviewed. Although experts did not rate any cases as having no support for the dosages for the entire medication regimen, in 11 of 24 cases the experts noted that the justification to support a particular dosage level was partially supported by the documentation. For example, experts found in 1 case with partially supporting documentation, that a child concurrently on seven different psychotropic medications received a dosage for an ADHD medication (Adderall) exceeding dosage guidelines based on FDA-approved or medical literature maximum dosages for children and adolescents.[19] Moreover, the documentation showed the child received a very small dose of an antipsychotic medication (quetiapine), suggesting that this agent was used for sleep, which experts said is not considered a good medical practice. In this case, the child was removed from the home at 14 months for, among other things, neglect and physical abuse.

Justification for Concurrent Use of Multiple Medications

Experts found that for 5 of 20 applicable cases, concurrent use of multiple psychotropic medications was mostly supported based on documentation. However, 14 of 20 cases included documentation that partially supported the concurrent use of multiple medications, and 1 case did not include any documentation to support concurrent use. For example, experts found in one case with partially supporting documentation that a toddler diagnosed with ADHD/oppositional defiant disorder and bipolar disorder was treated with complicated medication regimens, including mood stabilizers and antipsychotics, when other nonmedication interventions could have been considered, based on documentation reviewed. In this case the child was prescribed an ADHD medication (methylphenidate) and an antipsychotic medication (quetiapine) at 3-1/2 years of age. An ADHD medication (clonidine) and mood-stabilizing medication (oxcarbazepine) were tried by the time he was 4 years of age, and the child was maintained on as many as four psychotropic medications concurrently. As a 6-year-old, the child was treated with an antipsychotic (paliperidone) that has not been studied in children this age. There was limited discussion of potential risks or side effects though there were several reported adverse effects, including insomnia, agitation, and a possible movement disorder, potentially due to the use of antipsychotic medications, according to documentation reviewed.

Quality of Documentation to Support Informed and Shared Decision Making Varied among Selected Cases

For each of our cases, experts evaluated the foster and medical records for information related to informed and shared decision making— specifically, documentation of informed consent and communication between treatment providers. As shown in table 3, experts found that documentation to support informed consent and communication between treatment providers varied among selected cases reviewed.

Table 3. Quality of Documentation Support Related to Informed and Shared Decision Making

Category	Mostly supported in foster file or medical records	Partially supported in foster file or medical records	Not supported in foster file or medical records	Not applicable	Total applicablecases
Informed consent	5	11	7	1	23
Communication between treatment providers	15	5	3	1	23

Source: Expert reviewers.

Notes: The data are from expert reviews of foster file and medical records for 24 selected cases. Experts reviewed each of the categories from a quantitative and qualitative standpoint and provided their consensus evaluation based on documentation reviewed. The case selections include children prescribed a psychotropic drug as of 2008 and in foster care as of 2010 (nonrandomly selected infants did not have the 2010 restriction); however, the experts reviewed foster and medical information from the entire time the child was in foster care, which included the most-recent records available. Experts used the categorization "mostly supported in foster file or medical records" for instances where the documentation reviewed met both quantitative and qualitative measures as deemed appropriate by experts. Experts used the categorization "partially supported in foster file or medical records" for instances where the documentation included some information for the assessed category, but the documentation was either quantitatively or qualitatively, or both, lacking in some regard, according to experts. Experts used the categorization "not supported in foster file or medical records" for instances where there was no documentation for the assessed category, or the information provided was deemed substantively lacking by experts.

Informed Consent

Experts found that informed-consent decisions were mostly documented in 5 of 23 applicable cases. In 11 of 23 cases experts found partial documentation of informed consent—such as when some, but not all, medications prescribed to the child included documentation of informed consent—and 7 other cases did not include any documentation of informed consent. For example, in one case, experts reported there was no documentation of informed consent, psychiatric evaluation, psychiatric diagnosis, or monitoring of antipsychotic medication. In this case, the child was prescribed an antianxiety medication (buspirone), an antipsychotic medication (risperidone), and an ADHD medication (clonidine) at 4 years of age, presumably to treat psychiatric symptoms that interfered with his functioning, including short attention span, wandering off, self-injury, and aggression. However, experts noted the documentation was too sparse to determine why the psychotropic medications were prescribed, and the indications, monitoring, and side effects could not be evaluated.

Communication between Treatment Providers

Experts found that communication between treatment providers was mostly documented in 15 of 23 applicable cases. However, communication between treatment providers was partially documented in 5 of 23 cases, and there was no evidence that such communication occurred in 3 of 23 cases. For example, experts found in one case with partially supporting documentation that a teenage foster child with cognitive delays and fetal alcohol effects/exposure was diagnosed with ADHD and oppositional defiant disorder, and the quality of documentation showing communication between treatment providers varied by the child's placement setting. When the child was placed in a residential treatment facility, the communication between treatment providers was better documented than when the child was placed in a foster home. However, there was no clear documentation of communication between inpatient and outpatient providers and there was no clear evidence in the foster care files that the recommendations made by inpatient providers were actually provided as part of outpatient care.

Some Prescriptions in Infant Cases Were for Non-Mental-Health Reasons, but others Were for Psychiatric or Unclear Reasons

Of the 24 cases reviewed, 9 were infant cases that the experts evaluated to determine whether the prescriptions were for psychiatric or non-mentalhealth reasons.[20] Experts found in 4 of 9 infant cases reviewed that the prescription of psychotropic medication was for non-mental-health purposes, based on documentation reviewed. However, experts found that in 2 of 9 cases the infants were prescribed psychotropic medications for psychiatric reasons, and the rationale and oversight for such medications were partially supported by documentation. In 3 of 9 infant cases, experts were unable to discern whether the psychotropic medications were prescribed to infants for mental-health purposes or for some other medical reason, based on documentation reviewed. These results are summarized in table 4, below.

Table 4. Quality of Documentation Support Related to Infants Prescribed Psychotropic Medications

Category	Prescribed for non-mental-health purposes based on foster file and medical records	Prescribed for psychiatric purposes based on foster file and medical records	Not clear based on foster file or medical records	Total applicable cases
Infants prescribed psychotropic medications	4	2	3	9

Source: Expert reviewers.

Notes: Experts reviewed the case documentation from a quantitative and qualitative standpoint and provided their consensus evaluation. The infant cases selected included five infants less than 1 year of age prescribed any psychotropic medication during calendar year 2008 and in foster care as of January 2010. In addition, we also selected all children less than 1 year of age prescribed an ADHD, antipsychotic, or antidepressant medication during calendar year 2008, resulting in eight additional infant cases. However, we removed four of the cases from this review due to data-entry errors and potential Medicaid fraud, thus, a total of nine infant cases were reviewed. The experts reviewed foster and medical information from the entire time the child was in foster care, which included the most-recent records available.

Psychotropic Medications Prescribed to Infants for NonMental-Health Reasons

Experts found in two of nine infant cases that an antianxiety medication (hydroxyzine) was prescribed to treat skin conditions such as a rash and itchiness, and was not used for psychiatric purposes. In two other of nine other infant cases reviewed, an ADHD medication (clonidine) was used to treat sleep and irritability in children who had severe brain damage, and who by the clinical descriptions were inconsolable. For each of the above infant cases, experts agreed that there are no established standards for treating problems associated with devastating neurological impairment in infants. According to experts, although other medications, and possibly nonmedication interventions, could have been used instead of clonidine, the decision to treat was based on humanitarian reasons, and may have been necessary to maintain the child in the foster home given the marked distress displayed by the infants in these two cases. While physicians may use their discretion to prescribe these psychotropic medications to infants in these rare situations, non-mental-health uses still carry the same risk of adverse effects, including, for the ADHD medication clonidine, lowered blood pressure, changes in heart rate, and the potential for sudden death, and should therefore be carefully monitored.

Psychotropic Medications Prescribed to Infants for Psychiatric Reasons

Experts found in two of nine infant cases reviewed that the psychotropic medications were prescribed for psychiatric reasons, yet the justification for such prescriptions was not clear based on documentation. For example, experts found in one infant case that the child was prescribed an antidepressant (amitriptyline) at 9 months of age, and a prescription for an ADHD medication (clonidine) was added at 15 months of age to target complications of his neurological condition, including self-injurious behaviors, agitation, and aggression. Experts said there is no systematic research supporting the use of amitriptyline for self-injurious behaviors in any age group and the medication carries significant potential side effects, including cardiac side effects, and has been associated with sudden death in young children. Additionally, according to experts, amitriptyline can cause or exacerbate corneal ulceration, a painful condition for which this toddler was being treated, and which reportedly exacerbated the child's agitation. The case notes focus on medical issues with limited discussion of rationale, efficacy, or tolerability of psychotropic medications. In another infant case, experts found that clonidine was prescribed for sleep and behavioral issues, but the records did not show that the associated risks of the medications were discussed, and informed consent was not documented. According to experts, the medical records in this particular case also included a note from the prescribing doctor when the child was 20 months of age stating that clonidine was not a psychotropic medication while also stating that the medication was for behavioral problems.

Psychotropic Medications Prescribed to Infants for Unclear Reasons

Experts found in three of nine infant cases reviewed that documentation was unclear as to whether the psychotropic medications were prescribed for mental or non-mental-health purposes. For the first infant case with unclear documentation, experts noted that the child received a 2-month trial of an ADHD medication (clonidine) at 16 months of age, which experts stated they presumed was prescribed for irritability or difficulty sleeping, based on available documentation, but the actual indications were not documented. In the second infant case with unclear documentation, experts' review showed the child received a number of different anticonvulsants to try to improve seizure control. However, the infant was also prescribed a 2-month trial of an antianxiety medication (clonazepam) as a 1-year-old, and, according to the experts, the records did not indicate whether the medication was prescribed to treat the seizures or for psychiatric purposes. In the third infant case with unclear documentation, experts reported the child was prescribed an antianxiety medication (hydroxyzine), presumably to treat a skin irritation; however, there were no notes describing the rationale for the medication.

The experts agreed that prescriptions of psychotropic medications to infants carries significant risk as there are no established mental-health indications for the use of psychotropic medications in infants and the medications have the potential to result in serious adverse effects for this age group.

SELECTED STATES HAVE POLICIES AND PROCEDURES INTENDED TO ADDRESS OVERSIGHT OF PSYCHOTROPIC MEDICATIONS TO FOSTER CHILDREN, AND HHS ISSUED GUIDANCE FOR MONITORING PSYCHOTROPIC MEDICATIONS

Selected states have policies and procedures that are intended to provide oversight of psychotropic medications given to foster children. In addition, HHS has issued guidance, provided technical assistance, and facilitated information-sharing efforts among state child-welfare and Medicaid officials related to oversight of psychotropic medications for children in foster care. However, additional HHS guidance could help state child-welfare and

Medicaid officials manage psychotropic medications as states transition prescription drug benefits to managed care.

Selected States' Policies and Procedures Address Oversight of Psychotropic Medications to Foster Children

To varying degrees, each of the five selected states we reviewed has policies and procedures designed to address the monitoring and oversight of psychotropic medications prescribed to children in foster care. Some variation is expected because states set their own oversight guidelines. However, the 2011 Child and Family Services Improvement and Innovation Act required states to establish protocols for the appropriate use and monitoring of psychotropic medications prescribed to children in foster care, which ACF described in a 2012 program instruction.[21] According to ACF, the unique factors of each state, such as whether the child-welfare service-delivery structure is state- or county-administered, the type of Medicaid delivery system in place, and the availability of qualified practitioners, may influence how officials develop oversight protocols. Thus, according to ACF, each state needs to carefully assess existing oversight mechanisms and evaluate options in light of how they fit with the state's own set of needs and challenges. As part of ACF's 2012 program instructions, states are to address protocols for monitoring foster children's use of psychotropic medications as part of the state's APSR, which include protocols to address: (1) screening, assessment, and treatment planning mechanisms; (2) effective medication monitoring at both the client and the agency-wide level; and (3) shared decision making and communication among the prescriber, the child, caregivers, other health care providers, and the child-welfare worker.[22] Below are examples of selected states' policies and procedures—based on documents we reviewed and interviews with state Medicaid and child-welfare officials—that are intended to provide oversight of psychotropic medications to children in foster care. The information is presented using the same categories discussed above for experts' review of case studies. We did not assess the extent that these activities are being implemented effectively in the states.

Medical Pediatric Examinations

Each of our five selected states require that children in foster care receive medical examinations. For example, officials reported that in Oregon a child must receive a medical examination within 30 days and a mental-health exam within 60 days after the child enters the foster-care system, whereas Michigan officials said that both the medical and mental-health exams are to occur within 30 days.

Psychiatric Evaluations

All five selected states' foster-care programs use some type of functional assessment or screening tool, such as the Child and Adolescent Needs and Strengths (CANS), for screening and treatment planning, which may prompt a referral for a psychiatric evaluation as deemed appropriate. However, according to foster-care officials from Massachusetts, the CANS assessment tool is not sufficient to screen for a child's exposure to trauma and there is a need for a separate trauma-screening mechanism. Medicaid and foster-care officials from Texas told us in July 2013 that they are working to research and develop a comprehensive psychosocialassessment process with trauma screening/assessment components that is tailored to the unique needs of children in foster care. In April 2014, officials estimated that the process will take at least another year to implement and may be phased in so they could evaluate the effectiveness and refine the process.

Impact of Trauma Addressed by Treatment

Each of our five selected states has taken action to increase children's access to evidence-based therapies. For example, Oregon mental-health officials said that state law requires that 75 percent of the funding for mental-health agencies is to be used for evidence-based practices, and that the state surveys its mental health providers every 2 years on their utilization of evidence-based practices and reports these results to the state legislature. Oregon mental-health officials also said site reviews of mental-health providers occur every 3 years to make sure the providers are using practices on the state's approved list of evidence-based practices and if deficiencies are identified, correction plans are developed. As another example, Massachusetts's foster-care agency— through a federally funded grant—has provided evidence-based training on trauma-focused cognitive behavioral therapy, child-parent psychotherapy, and attachment self-regulation to both general practitioners and child-welfare staff to raise awareness and improve methods for treating and overseeing the child's overall health.

Each of our five selected states has taken action to improve focus on trauma-related needs of children in foster care. For example, Oregon was awarded a 3-year technical assistance grant by the Center for Health Care Strategies in April 2012. According to Oregon officials, one of the goals of this grant is to better understand the impact of trauma on emotions, behavior, and relationships, and to support training and policy development in this area. Beginning in May 2012, Texas implemented a 5-year strategic plan regarding trauma-informed care across the state for foster-care children. To do this, the state Medicaid program, foster-care agency, and managed-care organization (MCO) under contract are all working together to build a trauma-informed care system by incorporating trauma screening/assessment into psychosocial-assessment processes, enhancing clinical capacity to provide trauma-focused, evidence-based psychosocial therapy, training key stakeholders, and incorporating the principles of trauma-informed care into child-welfare policy and practices, according to Texas officials.

Prescriptions Appropriately Monitored

All five of the selected states have designed a mechanism to coordinate and share some or all Medicaid prescription claims data with the state's foster-care agency to help monitor and review cases based on varying criteria, such as prescriptions for children under a particular age, high dosages, or concurrent use of multiple medications. For example, according to Florida Medicaid officials, beginning in 2011 the state began requiring documentation of safety monitoring, such as metabolic monitoring, and body-mass-index information, to be included as part of the prior-authorization review process before particular medication regimens are approved for reimbursement.[23] However, these reviews are limited to those prescription claims paid for on a fee-for-service basis. Beginning in October 2014, foster children in Florida are to receive all of their Medicaid benefits through a third-party MCO, and it was unclear to state Medicaid officials how MCOs will provide oversight of psychotropic medications after the transition from fee-for-service to managed care occurs. Massachusetts uses both a fee-for-service model and MCOs to administer prescription claims benefits. Massachusetts child-welfare officials said that in the fee-for-service program, certain parameters, such as children in foster care prescribed four or more psychotropic medications, or two or more psychotropic medications of the same class, or children less than 6 years old prescribed a psychotropic medication, are flagged and forwarded to a child psychiatrist for additional review. However, among children served by MCOs, state Medicaid officials said that MCOs flag cases for children prescribed psychotropic drugs who are less than 6 years old, but state Medicaid officials were uncertain how MCOs followed up on these cases. In Texas there is a single MCO used to coordinate all prescription claims and medical services for children in foster care, and this organization works closely with the state foster-care agency to identify and monitor psychotropic medication use among children in foster care.

Appropriate Dosages Used

All five of the selected states have designed measures to review certain prescriptions that have dosages above a particular threshold. For example, in February 2005, Texas developed psychotropic drug-utilization parameters that outline what prescribing scenarios require an additional review, and these parameters were updated in January 2007, December 2010, and September 2013. Prescriptions that exceed usual recommended dosages for the child's age trigger an additional review from a child psychiatrist. Similarly, in 2012, Michigan's Medicaid and foster-care agencies began identifying and reviewing foster children's prescriptions if the medication exceeds the recommended dosages. According to officials, Florida, Massachusetts, and Texas Medicaid programs also require prior authorizations before a prescription is approved for reimbursement for various prescribing scenarios specific to psychotropic medications.[24] As stated in the section above concerning prescription monitoring, state Medicaid officials from Massachusetts and Florida told us they are still in the process of determining to what extent monitoring and oversight protocols—including prior authorizations— function for children in foster care who are prescribed medications through MCOs.

Justification for Concurrent Use of Multiple Medications

All five of the selected states have designed measures to review prescriptions for concurrent use of multiple medications to a varying extent. For example, the MCO that handles prescription claims for children in foster care in Texas monitors and completes additional reviews for concurrent prescriptions, and shares that information with the state foster-care and Medicaid agencies for the following medication regimens as stated in the September 2013 Texas Utilization parameters:

- four or more concurrent psychotropic medications;
- two or more concurrent antidepressants;
- two or more concurrent antipsychotic medications;

- two or more concurrent stimulant medications; and
- three or more concurrent mood-stabilizer medications.

Similarly, since 2012, the Michigan Medicaid agency monitors concurrent use of multiple medications using criteria, including four or more concurrent psychotropic medications, or two or more concurrent psychotropic medications within the same class, and shares this information with the state foster-care agency to facilitate additional reviews. Each of the above prescribing scenarios triggers an additional review that may include discussions with the prescriber to review the details and justification in support of the prescriptions. As mentioned previously in this report, Florida, Massachusetts, and Texas Medicaid programs also require prior authorizations before a prescription is approved for reimbursement for various prescribing scenarios specific to psychotropic medications. However, as stated above concerning prescription monitoring, state Medicaid officials from Massachusetts and Florida told us they are in the process of determining to what extent monitoring and oversight protocols—including prior authorizations— function for children in foster care prescribed medications through MCOs.

Informed Consent

Each of the five selected states require informed consent for psychotropic medications, but state practices vary. For example, according to agency officials, individuals authorized to give informed consent for a foster child vary across states. In Oregon, foster parents are not authorized to give informed consent for children in state custody—the foster child's case supervisor provides informed consent for psychotropic medications. As another example, officials from Texas told us that according to state law, when the court places a child in the custody of the state foster-care program, the court must authorize an individual or the child-welfare agency to consent to medical care for a child in foster care. When the court authorizes the child-welfare agency, the agency must designate a medical consenter—which typically includes emergency-shelter employees or live-in caregivers if the child is placed in community settings, or child-welfare staff when children are placed in facilities such as residential treatment centers.

Communication between Treatment Providers

Four of five selected states have some limitations regarding the extent to which a child's medical history is available to treatment providers. For example, in Oregon, medical providers have access to a child's prescription claims and medical history so long as the child was treated by a medical provider within the same Coordinated Care Organization (i.e., MCO), though the accessibility of information varies by each Coordinated Care Organization and is largely unavailable from competing Coordinated Care Organizations within the state. As another example, state Medicaid and foster-care officials from Michigan said they were in the process of developing electronic health records to improve access to information for prescribers, but noted that privacy concerns and legal limitations make it very difficult to share medical information across various medical providers. Texas is unique in that the state uses a single MCO to coordinate all prescription claims for children in foster care, which gives all participating medical providers access to prescription claims and the child's medical history electronically.

Psychotropic Prescriptions to Infants

Each of the five selected states, to varying extent, have designed measures to review prescriptions of psychotropic medications based on the child's age, which includes prescriptions to infants. For example, Oregon officials said that state law requires an annual review of medications by a licensed medical professional or qualified mental-health professional with authority to prescribe medications, other than the prescriber, if the child is covered by Medicaid and under the age of 6 years. Similarly, since 2012, Michigan's foster-care agency reviews medical records of all children in foster care less than 1 year old who are prescribed psychotropic medication to determine whether the prescription was for psychiatric purposes or non-mental-health reasons. As mentioned previously in this report, Florida, Massachusetts, and Texas Medicaid programs also require prior authorizations before a prescription is approved for reimbursement for various prescribing scenarios specific to psychotropic medications. Officials from Massachusetts and Florida told us they are in the process of determining how monitoring and oversight currently function for children in foster care who are prescribed medications through MCOs.

HHS Has Issued Guidance, Provided Technical Assistance, and Facilitated Information Sharing

In response to concerns and our December 2011 report recommendation related to the need for additional guidance for the prescribing of psychotropic medications for children in foster care, HHS's ACF has taken actions to improve the capacity of states' child-welfare agencies to effectively respond to the complex needs of children in foster care.[25] As previously mentioned in this report, ACF issued a program instruction in April 2012 to help states implement the new requirements in the Child and Family Services Improvement and Innovation Act regarding the development of protocols for oversight of psychotropic medication.[26] In addition, since our December 2011 report, ACF has worked collaboratively with CMS and SAMHSA to help states strengthen oversight of psychotropic medications to children in foster care by emphasizing the need for collaboration between state Medicaid, child-welfare, and mental-health officials in providing oversight; providing technical assistance; and facilitating information sharing.[27] Several initiatives were performed, including the following:

- CMS and SAMHSA participated in an ACF-led 2012 webinar series to help provide states with technical assistance in developing oversight and monitoring plans for psychotropic medications, as required by the Child and Family Services Improvement and Innovation Act. Using a question-and-answer format, the webinars featured experts, including researchers, child psychiatrists, and ACF staff, who provided ideas and feedback to state officials on planning efforts.

- In August 2012, ACF, CMS, and SAMHSA cohosted a conference for state child-welfare, Medicaid, and mental-health officials on strengthening the management of psychotropic medications for children in foster care. Conference sessions focused on effective collaborative medication monitoring, as well as creating data systems to facilitate collaboration, among other things. According to ACF, CMS, and SAMHSA officials, the conference was an opportunity for states to talk and share practices. According to ACF officials, representatives from 49 states attended, including officials from 4 of the 5 states covered by our review.[28] Officials from one of these states said the conference was beneficial. Officials from another state said participation challenged them to augment their system; officials from another state said it was helpful to hear what other states were doing; and officials from a fourth state said that it was important for the three federal agencies to have common goals, which would help sustain interagency collaboration at the state level.

In addition, CMS officials said the issue of psychotropic medications was a catalyst that caused the HHS agencies to look at broader issues related to mental health, including trauma-informed care and the use of mental-health screening tools and evidence-based therapies. ACF, CMS, and SAMHSA have undertaken several efforts, including the following:

- In 2012 and 2013, ACF announced funding opportunities for projects supporting the comprehensive use of evidence-based screening and assessment of mental and behavioral health needs, among other things.
- In March 2013, CMS issued guidance informing states about resources available to help meet the needs of children under the Early and Periodic Screening, Diagnostic, and Treatment (EPSDT) Medicaid benefit. Under the EPSDT, eligible individuals, such as children in foster care, are to be provided periodic screenings that include assessments of physical and mental-health development, as well as any medically necessary screenings to detect suspected illnesses or conditions not discovered during periodic exams. Results from screenings may trigger the need for further assessment to diagnose or treat a mental-health condition.
- In July 2013, ACF, CMS, and SAMHSA officials cosigned a letter to state child-welfare, Medicaid, and mental-health officials encouraging the integrated use of trauma-focused screening, functional assessments, and evidence-based practices to improve child well-being. In particular, federal officials noted that a high percentage of children in state foster care have been exposed to traumatic events and that there is reason to believe that problematic use of psychotropic medications is a reaction to the complexity of symptoms among children exposed to trauma and the lack of appropriate screening, assessment, and treatment.

Figure 1 below lists initiatives undertaken since our previous report by ACF, CMS, and SAHMSA.

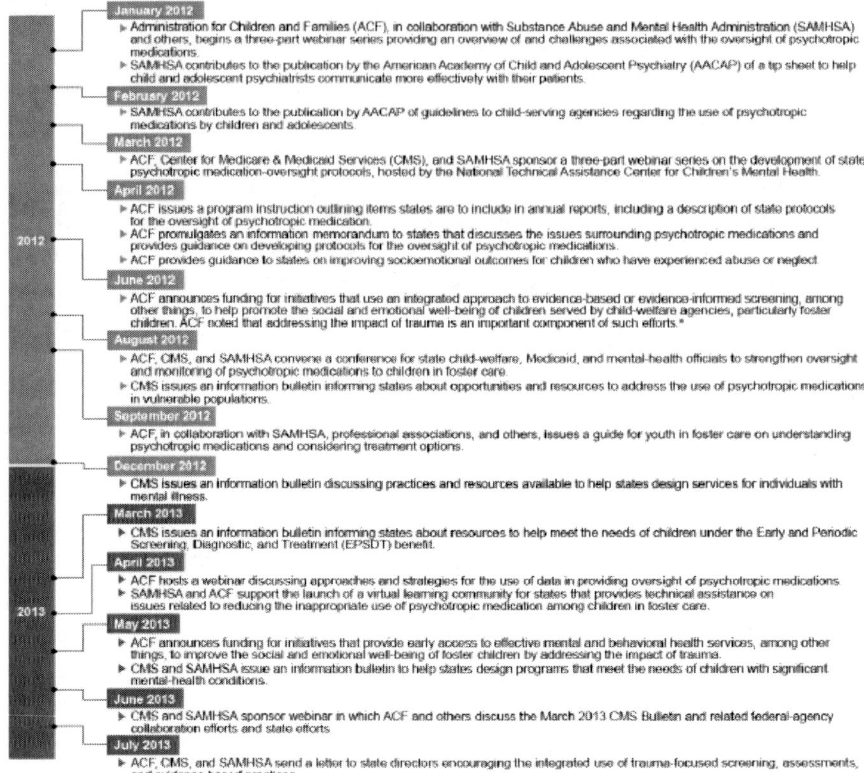

Source: GAO analysis of ACF, CMS, and SAMHSA documents and interviews.

[a]In June 2011, ACF announced the first of three recent funding initiatives focused on improving the social and emotional well-being of children in the child-welfare system by addressing the impact of trauma, among other things. The other two related funding initiatives were announced in June 2012 and May 2013.

Figure 1. Department of Health and Human Services (HHS) Efforts to Support States' Oversight of Psychotropic Medications among Children in Foster Care and Encourage the Use of Mental-Health Assessments and Screening Tools, since December 2011.

In addition, according to ACF officials, in collaboration with SAMHSA and others, ACF plans to issue guidance in August 2014 to foster parents regarding psychotropic medication to enhance their understanding of these medications.[29]

Additional Guidance Could Help Officials Manage Psychotropic Medications as States Transition Prescription-Drug Benefits to Managed Care

Three of five states included in our review use, or are transitioning from fee-for-service to, MCOs to administer prescription-drug benefits for mental-health medications; however, Medicaid officials from two of those three states reported that their states had conducted limited planning to ensure appropriate oversight of MCOs administering psychotropic medications—which creates a risk that state controls instituted in recent years under fee-for-service may not apply to managed care—and could benefit from additional federal guidance.

- In Massachusetts, most foster children receive drug benefits through fee-for-service, according to state Medicaid officials, though some children receive these benefits through MCOs.[30] Under fee-forservice, beginning in 2012, state Medicaid prescription claims data were to be provided to the state child-welfare agency to monitor and facilitate additional reviews, as necessary, for children prescribed medications in foster care. For example, according to child-welfare officials, cases that meet certain criteria—children less than 6 years old prescribed a psychotropic medication; children prescribed four or more psychotropic medications; or children prescribed two or more psychotropic medications in the same class—are flagged and forwarded to a child psychiatrist for further review. According to Massachusetts Medicaid officials, MCOs currently review cases when a child less than 6 years old is prescribed a psychotropic medication. State Medicaid officials said they did not know how MCOs followed up on cases last year. However, state Medicaid officials and other members of an interagency committee on psychotropic medications have met with MCO administrators to learn what they are doing to review cases and will continue to monitor MCOs, according to Massachusetts state officials.[31] Such operational information is important for the child-welfare agency to obtain to help ensure that appropriate oversight of psychotropic medication prescribed to foster children occurs. In addition, as part of the state's efforts to improve the prescribing, authorization, and monitoring of psychotropic medications, a Massachusetts interagency committee on psychotropic medications and foster children noted that MCOs' and the state's primary-care clinician plan program's role in the prior-authorization process has not been determined, in particular whether these organizations will have to assume responsibility for assuring that psychiatrists in their network adhere to the state's prescribing and monitoring practices.[32]

- Florida Medicaid officials said that beginning in 2014, MCOs will provide Medicaid participants, including foster children, with mental-health services, but it was unclear to state Medicaid officials how MCOs will provide oversight of psychotropic medications after the transition from fee-for-service to managed care occurs. Such operational information is also important for Florida's child-welfare agency to help ensure that appropriate oversight of psychotropic medication prescribed to foster children occurs. Florida Medicaid officials said that there will probably no longer be point-of-sale controls, which were instituted under fee-for-service in 2011. These controls, for example, required prescribers to submit forms indicating that safety monitoring, such as monitoring for signs of abnormal involuntary movement and metabolic monitoring, was performed for certain medications. If such point-of-sale controls are not continued under MCOs, then safety monitoring developed by the state under fee-for-service may not continue for children administered medications through MCOs.

ACF officials we met with noted that state child-welfare have experienced challenges coordinating with state Medicaid programs regarding the transition to MCOs, particularly with regard to data sharing. There are indications that the number of states using MCOs to administer drug benefits may increase. In 2012, the HHS Office of Inspector General (OIG) reported that 16 states used MCOs to administer drug benefits, and another 5 states had, or were planning, to switch to MCOs as a result of the Patient Protection and Affordable Care Act expansion of the Medicaid drug-rebate program, which allows states to obtain rebates from manufacturers for covered outpatient drugs.[33] Previously, medications dispensed by MCOs were excluded from such rebates.

According to *Standards for Internal Control in the Federal Government*, internal controls should generally be designed to assure that ongoing monitoring occurs in the course of normal operations, and is performed continually and ingrained in the agency's operations.[34] ACF requires states to develop effective medication monitoring at the agency and patient level. To this end, ACF, CMS, and SAMHSA have developed guidance for state Medicaid, child-welfare, and mental-health officials related to the oversight of psychotropic medications underscoring the need for collaboration between state officials to improve prescription monitoring. However, this guidance does not address oversight within the context of a managed-care environment, in which states rely on a third party to administer benefits such as psychotropic medications.[35] Additional guidance from HHS that helps states prepare and implement monitoring efforts within the context of a managed-care environment could help ensure appropriate oversight of psychotropic medications to children in foster care.

CONCLUSION

Since our December 2011 report, HHS has issued guidance regarding the oversight of psychotropic medications among children in foster care and has undertaken collaborative efforts to provide guidance and promote information sharing among states. In addition, HHS efforts have focused on using mental-health screening tools and providing therapies that address trauma, which seek to ensure that the mental-health needs of children in foster care are appropriately met. However, many states have, or are transitioning to, MCOs to administer prescription-drug benefits, and, as our work demonstrates, selected states have taken only limited steps to plan for the oversight of drug prescribing for foster children receiving health care through MCOs—which creates a risk that controls instituted in recent years under fee-for-service may not remain once states move to managed care. Additional guidance from HHS that helps states prepare and implement monitoring efforts within the context of a managed-care environment could help ensure appropriate oversight of psychotropic medications to children in foster care.

RECOMMENDATION FOR EXECUTIVE ACTION

To assist states that rely on or are planning to contract with an MCO to administer Medicaid prescription benefits, and to help provide effective oversight of psychotropic medications prescribed to children in foster care, we recommend that the Secretary of Health and Human Services issue guidance to state Medicaid, child-welfare, and mental-health officials regarding prescription-drug monitoring and oversight for children in foster care receiving psychotropic medications through MCOs.

AGENCY AND THIRD-PARTY COMMENTS AND OUR EVALUATION

We provided a draft copy of this report to HHS and the state foster-care and Medicaid agencies of the five selected states for their review. HHS, the Florida Agency for Health Care Administration, and the Massachusetts Executive Office of Health and Human Services provided written comments that are summarized below. HHS, Massachusetts, Oregon, and Texas provided technical comments, which we incorporated as appropriate. Michigan did not have any comments on the report.

In its response, HHS concurred with our recommendation to issue guidance to state Medicaid, child-welfare, and mental-health officials regarding prescription-drug monitoring and oversight for children in foster care receiving psychotropic medications through MCOs, and stated that CMS will work with other involved agencies to coordinate guidance between CMS and other HHS agencies. HHS further stated that guidance can be targeted regarding the use of MCOs for the foster-care population, but noted that previously issued guidance to state agencies from HHS already applies. However, the guidance that HHS referred to in its written comments is not specific to oversight within the context of a managed-care environment, and officials from the states in our review agreed that additional federal guidance could be beneficial. Therefore, we continue to believe that specific guidance to help states prepare and implement monitoring efforts within the context of a managed-care environment is needed to help ensure appropriate oversight of psychotropic medications to children in foster care.

In its written comments, the Florida Agency for Health Care Administration did not indicate whether it agreed or disagreed with our findings and recommendation, but said that it appreciated our efforts to evaluate Florida's Medicaid program and the reimbursement of psychotropic medications for foster children. Florida's response also provided additional information about the state's future plans for using managed-care plans and drug-utilization review requirements. For example, Florida's response stated that these managed-care plans must adhere to Florida statute requirements regarding prior-authorization procedures for covering medically necessary services, including prescription-drug services. However, the extent to which drug-utilization reviews and point-of-sale controls currently used by the state under feefor-service would apply after transitioning to MCOs is still unclear. For example, as we discussed in the report, if point-of-sale controls are not continued under MCOs, then safety monitoring developed by the state under fee-for-service may not continue for children administered medications through MCOs.

In its written comments, Massachusetts's Executive Office of Health and Human Services did not indicate whether it agreed or disagreed with our findings and recommendation, but thanked us for recognizing the work Massachusetts has done in the area of psychotropic medications being administered to children in foster care and agreed that discussion and investigation of this topic is timely and important to improve the health and welfare of children in foster care. In its response, Massachusetts noted that MCO contracts require the MCOs to monitor psychotropic prescribing for members under the age of 19 in accordance with guidelines established by Massachusetts's Psychoactive Medications in Children Working Group. Massachusetts also stated it conducted an operational review with each MCO to ensure that there is an established follow-up process for cases that are flagged, and that it continues to monitor MCOs closely to assure they remain in compliance with this contract requirement. However, the extent to which Massachusetts has developed guidelines, conducted operational reviews, and monitored for MCO compliance is still unclear.

Stephen M. Lord
Managing Director,
Forensic Audits and Investigative Service

APPENDIX I:
EXPERT SELECTION AND BIOGRAPHIES

To provide a clinical perspective on our cases, we contracted with two child psychiatrists who have clinical and research expertise in the use of psychotropic medications in children. We reviewed the curriculum vita for each expert who responded to our contract solicitation to determine whether the expert met all of the following criteria:

- is a medical doctor;
- is trained in child psychiatry;
- is board certified in child psychiatry;
- conducted relevant research or had relevant experience; and

- is a member of a relevant association (e.g., American Academy of Child and Adolescent Psychiatry).

We also conferred with officials from the National Institute of Mental Health.

We selected Jon McClellan, MD, and Michael Naylor, MD. Dr. McClellan is an attending psychiatrist at Seattle Children's Hospital; a professor at the University of Washington School of Medicine; and the medical director at Washington's Child Study and Treatment Center, the children's psychiatric hospital for the state of Washington. He is board certified in psychiatry and child and adolescent psychiatry, has conducted research regarding mental illness in children, and contributed to a forum on psychotropic medication use amongst children in foster care. Dr. Naylor is an associate professor at the University of Illinois at Chicago, School of Medicine, and the director of the Behavioral Health and Welfare Program, which was formed to address the mental-health needs of the most severely disturbed children in state care. He directs the Clinical Services in Psychopharmacology program, which provides an independent review of all psychotropic medication consent requests for foster children in Illinois. He is board certified in child and adolescent psychiatry, general psychiatry, and sleep-disorders medicine.

APPENDIX II:
CASE-RATING SUMMARY TABLE

The figure below contains the ratings assigned by experts for the quality and quantity of certain types of documentation contained in each child's foster and medical files. Cases are organized by the criteria used to randomly and nonrandomly select them and include reviews of cases from each of our selected states—Florida, Massachusetts, Michigan, Oregon, and Texas.

Figure 2 — Case-Rating Summary Table.

Foster Child

Randomly selected from each state (columns 1–18):
- A child prescribed any psychotropic medication during calendar year 2008 — columns 1–4
- A child with prescriptions exceeding dosage guidelines developed by the state of Texas, based on medical literature and FDA-approved maximum dosages — columns 5–9
- A child prescribed five or more medications concurrently — columns 10–14
- A child less than 1 year of age prescribed any psychotropic medication — columns 15–18

Nonrandomly selected from each state (columns 19–24):
- Any child less than 1 year old prescribed an attention deficit hyperactivity disorder (ADHD) medication, antipsychotic, or antidepressant — columns 19–24

	1	2	3	4	5	6	7	8	9	10	11	12	13	14	15	16	17	18	19	20	21	22	23	24	Total (Mostly)	Total (Partially)	Total (Not)	Total (N/A)
Medical pediatric examinations																									22	2	0	0
Psychiatric evaluations											N/A		N/A		N/A	N/A	N/A	N/A	N/A						12	3	2	7
Evidence-based therapies provided											N/A	N/A	N/A	N/A	N/A	N/A	N/A	N/A	N/A						3	11	1	9
Impact of trauma addressed by treatment	N/A								N/A		N/A	N/A	N/A		N/A	N/A	N/A	N/A	N/A						3	8	3	10
Prescriptions appropriately monitored																									13	9	2	0
Appropriate dosages used																									13	11	0	0
If used, was concurrent use justified											N/A		N/A		N/A					N/A					5	14	1	4
Informed consent obtained											N/A														5	11	7	1
Communication between treatment providers											N/A														15	5	3	1
Psychiatric diagnosis fit history																									12	11	1	0
Prescriptions indicated for diagnostic status																									17	6	1	0
Duration of trials adequate																									23	0	1	0
Medication increases or changes systematic																									21	3	0	0
Ongoing efficacy evaluated																									14	7	3	0
Psychosocial services provided													N/A												22	1	0	1
Total (Mostly):	12	7	4	5	8	11	8	7	8	7	8	10	8	5	8	11	12	12	6	11	11	4	11	6				
Total (Partially):	2	8	10	7	7	3	7	1	5	8	0	1	1	3	4	0	0	0	6	3	4	9	4	9				
Total (Not):	0	0	1	3	0	1	0	7	1	0	0	2	2	6	0	0	0	0	0	0	0	2	0	0				
Total (N/A):	1	0	0	0	0	0	0	0	1	0	7	2	4	1	3	4	3	3	3	1	0	0	0	0				

Legend:
- Mostly supported in foster file or medical records
- Partially supported in foster file or medical records
- Not supported in foster file or medical records
- N/A — Not applicable

Source: Expert reviewers.

Notes: The data are from expert reviews of foster file and medical records for 24 selected cases. Experts reviewed each of the categories from a quantitative and qualitative standpoint and provided their consensus evaluation based on documentation reviewed. The case selections include children prescribed a psychotropic drug as of 2008 and in foster care as of 2010 (nonrandomly selected infants did not have the 2010 restriction); however, the experts reviewed foster and medical information from the entire time the child was in foster care, which included the most-recent records available. Experts used the categorization "mostly supported in foster file or medical records" for instances where the documentation reviewed met both quantitative and qualitative measures as deemed appropriate by experts. Experts used the categorization "partially supported in foster file or medical records" for instances where the documentation included some information for the assessed category, but the documentation was either quantitatively or qualitatively, or both, lacking in some regard, according to experts. Experts used the categorization "not supported in foster file or medical records" for instances where there was no documentation for the assessed category, or the information provided was deemed substantively lacking by experts.

Figure 2. Case-Rating Summary Table.

End Notes

[1] GAO, Foster Children: HHS Guidance Could Help States Improve Oversight of Psychotropic Prescriptions, GAO-12-201 (Washington, D.C.: Dec. 14, 2011); Children's Mental Health: Concerns Remain about Appropriate Services for Children in Medicaid and Foster Care, GAO-13-15 (Washington, D.C.: Dec. 10, 2012).

[2] Off-label use refers to the prescription of a medication for uses other than what the Food and Drug Administration (FDA) has approved. Medicaid Medical Directors Learning Network and Rutgers Center for Education and Research on Mental Health Therapeutics, Antipsychotic Medication Use in Medicaid Children and Adolescents: Report and Resource Guide from a 16-State Study (New Brunswick, N.J.: July 2010).

[3] GAO-12-201. We initially selected six states—Florida, Maryland, Massachusetts, Michigan, Oregon, and Texas—that had a fee-for-service Medicaid prescription program, reflected a range of geographic diversity, and included large and small populations of children in foster care. However, Maryland's 2008 foster care data were determined to be unreliable for the purposes of our previous work, so that state was excluded from our December 2011 report and is not part of this review.

[4] Analysis included in our December 2011 report used dosage guidelines developed by the state of Texas based on FDA-approved or medical literature maximum dosages for children and adolescents. ACF lists these guidelines as an example for other states. For additional information, see GAO-12-201 and Texas Department of Family and Protective Services, and the University of Texas at Austin College of Pharmacy, Psychotropic Medication Utilization Parameters for Foster Children (Austin, Tex.: December 2010).

[5] American Academy of Child and Adolescent Psychiatry, A Guide for Community Child Serving Agencies on Psychotropic Medications for Children and Adolescents (Feb. 12, 2012).

[6] The case studies selected for this review were taken from the data used in our December 2011 report, GAO-12-201. For the randomly selected cases, we selected from the population of children who were still in foster care as of January 2010. This date was used as it was the date of the most-recent enrollment data of children in foster care across all five states. The date requirement effectively sets a minimum amount of time the child is in foster care, which could skew our selection towards children with greater mental-health needs, as children who stay in foster care longer tend to be older and have more medications. Once the cases were selected, experts reviewed foster and medical information spanning the entire time the child was in foster care, which included the most-recent records available.

[7] For each of these cases, we asked state officials to review the child's records and confirm the child had not received a psychotropic medication.

[8] Experts used the categorization "not applicable" for instances where the category did not apply to the child's case, such as an infant prescribed a psychotropic drug for non-mentalhealth reasons.

[9] State officials noted that in some circumstances that additional medical documents may exist, but these documents were not located and provided to GAO as requested.

[10] GAO, Standards for Internal Control in the Federal Government, GAO/AIMD-00-21.3.1 (Washington, D.C.: November 1999).

[11] Child and Family Services Improvement and Innovation Act, Pub. L. No. 112-34, § 101(b)(1) and (2), 125 Stat. 369 (amending 42 U.S.C. § 622(b)(15)(A)).

[12] See U.S. Department of Health and Human Services, Administration for Children and Families, Program Instruction, ACYF-CB-PI-12-05 (Washington, D.C.: Apr. 11, 2012).

[13] GAO-12-201.

[14] GAO-12-201.

[15] Other categories reviewed that related to screening, assessment, and treatment planning include "psychosocial services provided" and "diagnosis fits history" and are shown in app. II.

[16] Schizotypal disorder is a condition in which an individual has disturbances in thought patterns, appearance, and behavior, among other things.

[17] Medication dose amounts were compared by experts to guidelines developed by the state of Texas, which are based on FDA approved or medical literature maximum dosages. For additional information see Texas Department of Family and Protective Services, and the University of Texas at Austin College of Pharmacy, Psychotropic Medication Utilization Parameters for Foster Children.

[18] Other categories reviewed related to medication monitoring include "prescriptions indicated for diagnostic status," "duration of trials adequate," "ongoing efficacy evaluated," and "medication increases or changes systematic" and are shown in app. II.

[19] Medication dose amounts were compared by experts to guidelines developed by the state of Texas, which are based on FDA approved or medical literature maximum dosages. For additional information see Texas Department of Family and Protective Services, and the University of Texas at Austin College of Pharmacy, Psychotropic Medication Utilization Parameters for Foster Children (Austin, Tex.: December 2010).

[20] The infant cases selected included five infants less than 1 year of age prescribed any psychotropic medication during calendar year 2008 and in foster care as of January 2010. In addition, we also selected all children less than 1 year of age prescribed an ADHD, antipsychotic, or antidepressant medication during calendar year 2008, resulting in eight additional infant cases. However, we removed four of the cases from this review due to data-entry errors and potential Medicaid fraud, thus, a total of nine infant cases were reviewed. Because the experts reviewed foster and medical records spanning the entire period the child was in foster care, in some infant cases the medication regimens reviewed go beyond the child's infancy. To the extent possible, the specific age of the child when the medication was prescribed is noted. To determine the categorizations of whether the medications were provided for mental- or non-mental-health reasons, we considered the experts' review of infant cases for up to 2 years of age.

[21] Child and Family Services Improvement and Innovation Act, Pub. L. No. 112-34, § 101(b)(2), 125 Stat. 369 (2011). See Administration for Children and Families, Program Instruction, ACYF-CB-PI-12-05.

[22] See Administration for Children and Families, Program Instruction, ACYF-CB-PI-12-05.

[23] Medication regimens that require prior authorization include antipsychotic prescriptions that exceed a particular dosage, and antipsychotic or antidepressant medications prescribed to a child less than 6 years old.

[24] For example, we were told that Florida requires prior authorization for children ages 6-17 years who are prescribed a high-dose antipsychotic medication, and Texas has dosage requirements for some antidepressants. Massachusetts reportedly has prior-authorization requirements for certain psychotropic drugs, such as antipsychotic medications. Officials explained that state law restricts Oregon and Michigan's ability to conduct prior authorizations at the point of sale for behavioral-health medications generally.

[25] GAO-12-201.

[26] See Administration for Children and Families, Program Instruction, ACYF-CB-PI-12-05.

[27] In November 2011, shortly before our previous report was issued, ACF, CMS, and SAMHSA officials cosigned a letter to the directors of state child-welfare, Medicaid, and mental-

health agencies outlining the actions each division was taking to support state efforts to strengthen psychotropic prescription oversight. In addition, the letter also noted that it is essential for state child-welfare, Medicaid, and mental-health officials to collaborate, particularly in efforts to improve medication use and prescription monitoring.

[28] A Florida child-welfare official said that Florida officials were unable to attend the conference due to a hurricane.

[29] In addition, the President's fiscal year 2015 budget submission proposes a new Medicaid demonstration project in partnership with ACF to encourage states to provide evidence-based psychosocial interventions to children and youth in foster care.

[30] As part of our December 2011 report, we analyzed Medicaid claims data for 2008 and determined that about 72 percent of foster children in Massachusetts received drug benefits through fee-for-service. In the fall of 2013, Massachusetts Medicaid officials confirmed that most children in foster care continue to receive drug benefits through feefor-service.

[31] Formed in 2007, the Psychoactive Medications in Children Working Group comprises MassHealth, the Massachusetts Department of Mental Health, and the Massachusetts Department of Children and Families, among others, and works to evaluate and recommend strategies to improve psychoactive medication management in children served by MassHealth.

[32] Formed in 2012, the Steering Committee for Monitoring Psychotropic Medications for Children in Foster Care was charged with developing a plan to promote best practices related to the prescription, authorization, and monitoring of psychotropic medications. The committee is led by the Massachusetts Child Advocate and the Department of Children and Families Commissioner. According to Massachusetts officials, the committee has developed a proposed initiative that would require prior authorization on combinations of medications that have little or no evidence of safe and effective use in the very young as well as situations identified as polypharmacy.

[33] Department of Health and Human Services, Office of Inspector General, States' Collection of Rebates for Drugs Paid Through Medicaid Managed Care Organizations, OEI-03-11-00480 (September 2012); Pub. L. No. 111-148, § 2501(c), 124 Stat. 119, 308 (2010).

[34] GAO, Standards for Internal Control in the Federal Government, GAO/AIMD-00-21.3.1 (Washington, D.C.: November 1999).

[35] CMS has made tools available on its website to help states design programs to manage MCO quality.

In: Psychotropic Medication …   ISBN: 978-1-63485-155-8
Editor: Malcolm C. Burgess   © 2016 Nova Science Publishers, Inc.

Chapter 3

PROMOTING THE SAFE, APPROPRIATE, AND EFFECTIVE USE OF PSYCHOTROPIC MEDICATION FOR CHILDREN IN FOSTER CARE[*]

Administration for Children and Families

INFORMATION MEMORANDUM

To: State, Tribal and Territorial Agencies Administering or Supervising the Administration of Titles IV-B and IV-E of the Social Security Act, Indian Tribes and Indian Tribal Organizations

Subject: Promoting the Safe, Appropriate, and Effective Use of Psychotropic Medication for Children in Foster Care

Purpose: To serve as a resource to State and Tribal title IV-B agencies as they comply with requirements to develop protocols for the appropriate use and monitoring of psychotropic medications in the title IV-B plan. This Information Memorandum (IM) defines the issues surrounding psychotropic medication use by children in foster care, highlights available resources for States to consider when developing their Annual Progress and Services Report (APSR), and encourages increasing access to clinically appropriate screening,

---

[*] This information memorandum (ACYF-CB-IM-12-03) was published by the Adminstration on Children, Youth and Families, Administration for Children and Families, U.S. Department of Health and Human Services, April 11, 2012.

assessment, and evidence-based interventions for foster children with mental health and trauma-related needs.

Legal and Related References: Section 422(b)(15) of the Social Security Act (the Act)

Statutory Background: Recent statutory mandates require States, Territories and Tribes that administer title IV-B, subpart 1 programs to address some of the most pressing issues related to psychotropic medication prescription oversight and monitoring for children in foster care. These include:

- The *Fostering Connections to Success and Increasing Adoptions Act of 2008* (Public Law (P.L.) 110-351) amended title IV-B, subpart 1 of the Social Security act to require State and Tribal[1] title IV-B agencies to develop a plan for ongoing oversight and coordination of health care services for children in foster care, in coordination and consultation with the State title XIX (Medicaid) agency, pediatricians, and other experts in health care, as well as experts in and recipients of child welfare services. The plan must describe how it will ensure a coordinated strategy to identify and respond to the health care needs of children in foster care placements, including mental health and dental health needs, and provide for continuity of health care services, which may include establishing a "medical home" for children who are in foster care. The purpose of these requirements is to ensure that children in foster care receive high-quality, coordinated health care services, including appropriate oversight of any needed prescription medicines (section 422(b)(15) of the Act).

- The *Child and Family Services Improvement and Innovation Act* (P.L. 112-34) amended the law by adding to the requirements for the health care oversight and coordination plan. Whereas the law had previously required that the plan address "oversight of prescription medicines," the new provision builds on this requirement by specifying that the plan must include an outline of "protocols for the appropriate use and monitoring of psychotropic medications." In addition, P.L. 112-34 requires that the health care oversight and coordination plan outline "how health needs identified through screenings will be monitored and treated, including emotional trauma associated with a child's maltreatment and removal from home" (section 422(b)(15)(A) of the Act).

Although not initially mandated by statute, it should be noted that the Children's Bureau (CB) has always encouraged title IV-B agencies to address oversight of psychotropic medications in the plan for ongoing oversight and coordination of health care services since the first guidance on the health care plan was issued in 2009 (see ACYF-CB-PI-09-06 and ACYF-CB-09-07). With the amendments made by P.L. 112-34, it is now a statutory requirement that oversight of psychotropic medications be explicitly addressed in the health care oversight and coordination plan.

States and Tribes will need to address how they are responding to these new requirements in their Annual Progress and Services Reports (APSRs) which are due on June 30, 2012.

Issue Background:

Prevalence of Psychotropic Medication Use Among Children in Foster Care

There has been a steady rise in the use of medication to address children's emotional and behavioral problems over the last decade, even among pre-schoolers.[2] For example, one study found that, in 1996, approximately four percent of youth in the general population received psychotropic medication: almost three times the usage rates reported in 1987.[3]

At this time, there is no comprehensive source of data regarding psychotropic medication usage rates for children and adolescents in child welfare, including data on those in foster care. Rather, existing data: 1) is not current, lagging behind by as much as a decade; 2) is often geographically specific (e.g., from one State); and 3) comes from research conducted on the broader population of children who are involved with child welfare agencies (including children served in their own homes, as well as children who are in foster care). Despite these deficiencies, published studies consistently reveal even higher rates of use for children involved in child welfare than in the general population, with usage rates between 13 and 52 percent.[4,5,6,7,8,9,10] Moreover, studies have shown the following with regard to the prevalence of psychotropic drug use and factors influencing the likelihood of use among children in foster care:[11]

- *Age* : Children in foster care are more likely to be prescribed psychotropic medications as they grow older, with 3.6 percent of two to five year-olds taking psychotropic medication at a given time. This increases to 16.4 percent of 6-11 year olds and 21.6 percent of 12- 16 year olds. The likelihood that a child will be prescribed multiple psychotropic medications also increases with age.

- *Gender*: Males in foster care are more likely to be receiving psychotropic medications (19.6 percent) than their female counterparts (7.7 percent).

- *Behavioral Concerns:* Children scoring in the clinical range on the Child Behavioral Checklist, a common tool for assessing both internalizing and externalizing behavioral issues among children and youth, are much more likely than those with subclinical scores to receive psychotropic medications.

- *Placement Type:* Children in the most restrictive placement setting are the most likely to receive psychotropic medications. In group or residential homes, nearly half of the young people are taking at least one psychotropic drug. Additionally, children in more restrictive placement types are more likely to be taking multiple psychotropic medications.

- *Geographic Variation:* There are also significant geographic variations within and across States in the prevalence of psychotropic use among children in foster care. These varying rates of use cannot be attributed to population differences, suggesting that factors other than clinical need may be influencing the practice of prescribing psychotropic medications.[12] In a national study, rates of medication use varied 0-40 percent, representing a 40-fold variation across catchment areas.[13] It should be noted, however, that while these data raise concerns about medication overuse, there is also data to suggest that some foster children (e.g., those in rural areas) may actually be prescribed at lower than normal rates and this suggests they may not have adequate access to needed psychiatric care.[14]

Social-Emotional, Behavioral, and Mental Health Needs of Children with Child Welfare Involvement

- Children who come to the attention of the child welfare system have disproportionally high rates of social-emotional, behavioral, and mental health challenges.[15] These social-emotional, behavioral and mental health concerns include the following:

- 23 percent of children age 17 and under who have experienced maltreatment have behavior problems requiring clinical intervention. Clinical-level behavior problems are almost three times as common among this population as among the general population. Both internalizing problems (e.g., depression, anxiety, being withdrawn) and externalizing problems (e.g., aggression, delinquency) are common in children who have experienced maltreatment. Among children who enter foster care, approximately one third scored in the clinical range for behavior problems on the Child Behavior Checklist.
- 35 percent of children age 17 and under who have experienced maltreatment demonstrate clinical-level problems with social skills – more than twice the rate of the general population.
- Children in foster care are more likely to have a mental health diagnosis than other children. In a study of foster youth between the ages of 14 and 17, [16] 63 percent met the criteria for at least one mental health diagnosis at some point in their life. The most common diagnoses were Oppositional Defiant Disorder/Conduct Disorder, Major Depressive Disorder/Major Depressive Episode, Attention Deficit/Hyperactivity Disorder, and Posttraumatic Stress Disorder.
- According to one study, by the time they are age 17, 62 percent of youth in foster care will exhibit both the symptoms of a mental health disorder and the symptoms of trauma.[17]
- Although they make up only three percent of the Medicaid population under age 18, children in foster care account for 32 percent of the recipients of behavioral health services in this age group.[18]

These data clearly show that the broader group of children who experience maltreatment and come to the attention of a child welfare agency (of which children in foster care are a subset) have emotional and behavioral problems that derail normal development, hinder healthy functioning, and impede the achievement of permanency.

Appropriateness of Psychotropic Medication Use Among Children in Foster Care

Although numerous studies have demonstrated that the rates of psychotropic medication prescriptions are high among children in foster care, these rates, at least in part, may reflect increased levels of emotional and behavioral distress. Figure I (below) demonstrates the high level of mental health needs among children involved with the child welfare system and illustrates the relationship between the clinical need and the use of psychotropic medications across three age groups. In addition, Figure 2 shows that, with the exception of residential treatment settings, the rate of psychotropic medication prescription is relatively consistent regardless of whether children were served in their own homes or removed from the home and placed in either kinship care or a foster family home; suggesting that rates of mental health needs and associated use of psychotropic medications are not primarily the result of removing children from their homes.

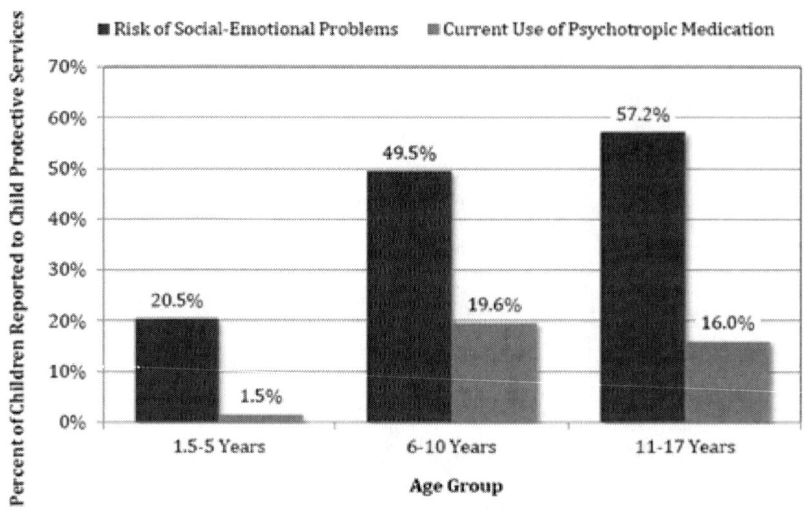

Data Source: National Survey of Child and Adolescent Well-Being II (NSCAW II). NSCAW II is a Congressionally required study sponsored by the Office of Planning, Research and Evaluation, Administration for Children and Families (ACF), U.S. Department of Health and Human Services (DHHS).

Risk of social-emotional problems was defined as scores in the clinical range on any of the following standardized measures: Internalizing, Externalizing or Total Problems scales of the Child Behavior Checklist (CBCL: administered for children 1.5 to 18 years old), Youth Self Report (YSR; administered to children 11 years old and older), or the Teacher Report From (TRF; administered for children 6 to 18 years old); the Child Depression Inventory (CDI; administered to children 7 years old and older); or the PTSD section Intrusive Experiences and Dissociation subscales of the Trauma Symptoms Checklist (administered to children 8 years old and older).

Figure 1. Risk of Social-Emotional Problems and Use of Psychotropic Medications among Children Known to Child Welfare, by Age Group.

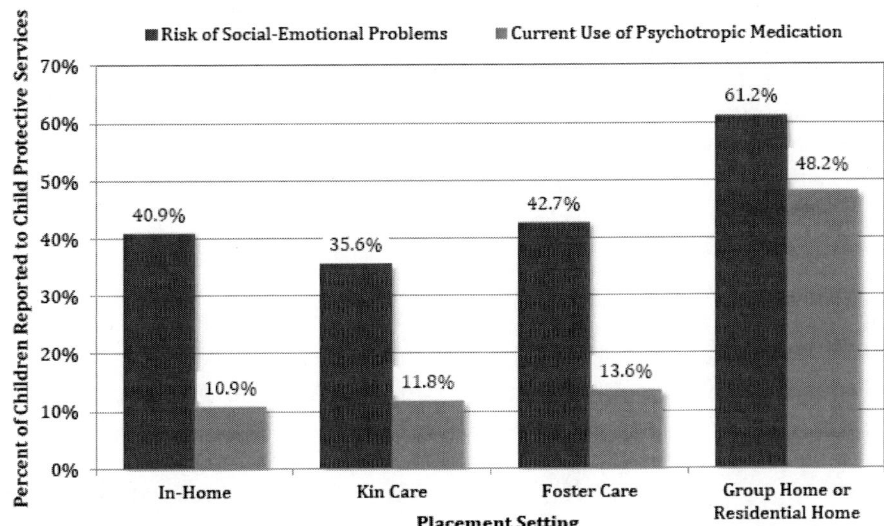

Data Source: National Survey of Child and Adolescent Well-Being II (NSCAW II). NSCAW II is a Congressionally required study sponsored by the Office of Planning, Research and Evaluation, Administration for Children and Families (ACF), U.S. Department of Health and Human Services (DHHS).

Risk of social-emotional problems was defined as scores in the clinical range on any of the following standardized measures: Internalizing, Externalizing or Total Problems scales of the Child Behavior Checklist (CBCL: administered for children 1.5 to 18 years old), Youth Self Report (YSR; administered to children 11 years old and older), or the Teacher Report From (TRF; administered for children 6 to 18 years old); the Child Depression Inventory (CDI; administered to children 7 years old and older); or the PTSD section Intrusive Experiences and Dissociation subscales of the Trauma Symptoms Checklist (administered to children 8 years old and older).

Figure 2. Risk of Social-Emotional Problems and Use of Psychotropic Medications among Children Known to Child Welfare, by Placement Type.

The graphics above demonstrate that many children in foster care have mental health challenges requiring intervention, which may include the appropriate use of psychopharmacological treatments as part of a comprehensive treatment approach. Unfortunately, research on the safe and appropriate pediatric use of psychotropic medications lags behind prescribing trends.[19] There is even less evidence of the effectiveness of pharmacologic interventions for the treatment of trauma-related symptoms in children.[20] In the absence of such research, it is not possible to know all of the short- and long-term effects, both positive and negative, of psychotropic medications on young minds and bodies.

Patterns that may signal that factors other than clinical need are impacting the prescription of psychotropic medications are referred to as "outlier practices" or "red flags." Practices that may be of concern include instances where children are prescribed too many psychotropic medications, too much medication, or at too young an age: too many, and too much, too young.

- Too many: Children with histories of maltreatment, including those in foster care, often present with complex trauma-related and mental health needs, often demonstrating multiple diagnoses at one time (i.e., co-morbidity). To treat the multiple mental and behavioral health symptoms that a child may exhibit, more than one drug – and often more than one type of medication–are prescribed. There is, however, scant evidence of the effectiveness of using multiple psychotropic medications at once (polypharmacy). No research supports the use of five or more psychotropic drugs.

  Despite the lack of supporting evidence and the potential for adverse effects (e.g., side effects, drug interactions, metabolic effects, and potential that some medications may alter nervous system development), polypharmacy is on the rise. A 2002 study of children in the general population showed an increase of greater than 600 percent (0.03 per 100 to 0.23) in the rate of prescription of more than one psychotropic medication at a time.21 A 2008 study of children in foster care taking psychotropic medication found 21.3 percent are receiving mono-therapy (one class of psychotropic medication), 41.3 percent are taking three or more classes of psychotropic medications, 15.4 percent are taking medication from four or more classes, and 2.1 percent are taking five or more classes of psychotropic drugs.22 These trends are further reflected in data from the National Survey of Child and Adolescent Well-Being, which shows the proportion of children reported to child protective services who are receiving two or more psychotropic medications at once (see Figure 3 below).

Prescription patterns that may be of concern in this category include: children taking three or more medications at a time; prescription of two or more medications in the same class for more than 30 days, and prescribing multiple psychotropic medications before testing the effectiveness of a single medication (polypharmacy before monopharmacy).

- Too Much: Another potential outlier practice or "red flag" that may be cause for concern is prescriptions in dosages that exceed recommendations. Because very few psychotropic medications are tested on children, research-based guidelines for medication dosages exist for very few psychotropic medications prescribed to children. Prescription labeling by the Food and Drug Administration (FDA) is one way that dosage guidelines are established, however, the majority of pediatric psychotropic use is off-label. This means that even though the drug can legally be used, the product label does not specify that it was approved for a particular age group or particular treatment application. [24]

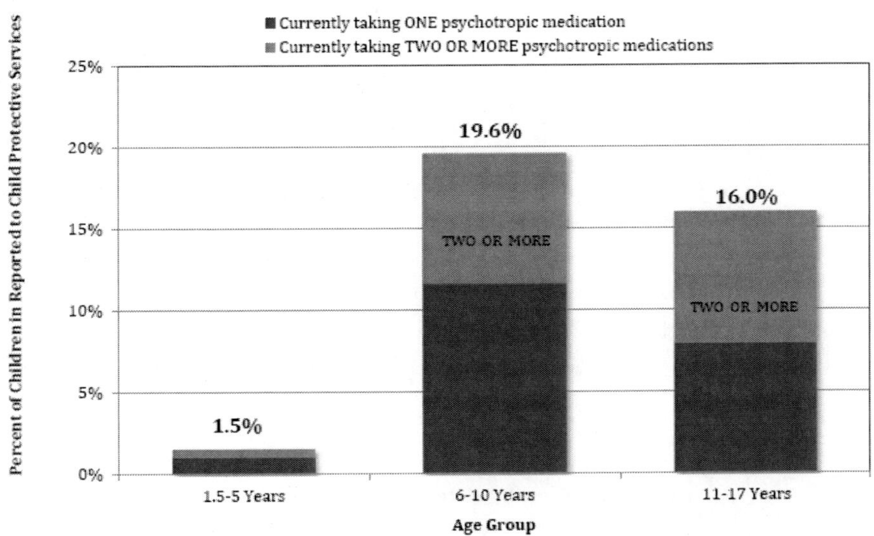

Data Source: National Survey of Child and Adolescent Well-Being II (NSCAW II). NSCAW II is a Congressionally required study sponsored by the Office of Planning, Research and Evaluation, Administration for Children and Families (ACF), U.S. Department of Health and Human Services (DHHS).

Figure 3. Psychotropic Medication Use and Polypharmacy among Children Known to Child Welfare, by Age Group.

In the absence of a robust research base and evidence-based prescription guidelines, some jurisdictions have adopted consensus-based approaches that attempt to define safe and effective use of psychotropic medications for a variety of mental health diagnoses found in children and adolescents. One such set of practice parameters was developed by the State of Texas, with guidance from an expert panel, to be used as a resource for physicians and other clinicians.[25] Other States have implemented systems that require prior authorization and, in some cases, mandatory second opinions in an effort to ensure appropriate use of psychotropic medication for foster children (including proper dosage).[26]

Until all drugs are properly studied in the populations for which they are being used, the lack of specific evidence-based recommendations reinforces the need for close supervision and monitoring for patients receiving psychotropic medication for off-label uses.[27]

- Too Young: According to a study by Zito and colleagues (2000), between 1991-1995 there was a 50 percent increase in the rate at which preschool children (age 2-4) were prescribed psychotropic medications, with 1.5 percent of preschoolers being prescribed stimulants or other psychotropic medication.[28] A 2011 report from a Government Accountability Office (GAO) examining psychotropic use in five states found foster children have higher rates of psychotropic use than other children enrolled in the Medicaid program.[29] Specifically, the GAO study found that 0.3 to 2.1 percent of children in foster care under one year old were prescribed potentially psycho-active medications (most commonly antihistamines and benzodiazepines) compared to a 0.1 to 1.2 percent of children not in foster care.

  Psychotropic medication use with young children is of special concern since this population may be especially vulnerable to adverse effects, necessitating careful management and oversight.[30]

Beyond "too many, too much, too young", the dramatic increase in the use of antipsychotic medication for children and adolescents over the past two decades has also raised concern. While prescription rates have risen across-the-board, a recent 16-State study found that foster children received antipsychotic medications at a rate almost nine times that of other children covered by Medicaid even though they represent only three percent of those covered. [31] Although this study was not able to explicitly examine the relationship between mental health diagnosis and prescribing patterns, other published research suggests that psychotropic drugs are being overused to manage emotional problems and disruptive behavior that might better be addressed by non-pharmacological treatment approaches.

When used appropriately, antipsychotic medications may provide a legitimate treatment option for some children in foster care. However, it is generally recommended that prescription of antipsychotic medications be closely monitored, especially when they are prescribed for more than two years and when they are used without a diagnosis of schizophrenia, bipolar disorder, or psychosis.

In summary, while medication can be an important component of a comprehensive response to the complex mental health needs of children in foster care, current use of psychotropic medications among children in foster care at times may exceed practice standards that are supported by empirical research. The following factors may play a role in these patterns of psychotropic medication use in foster children:[32]

- Insufficient State oversight and monitoring of psychotropic medication use;

- Gaps in coordination and continuity of medical and mental health care across public health and social service systems involved with affected children and their families;

- Provider shortages, especially of board-eligible and board-certified child and adolescent psychiatrists, in some geographic areas (e.g., rural areas); and

- Lack of access to effective non-pharmacological treatments in outpatient settings.

Strengthened oversight of psychotropic medication use is necessary in order to responsibly and effectively attend to the clinical needs of children who have experienced maltreatment. The processes and practices suggested by this document provide increased opportunities for that oversight for children in foster care.

Practice Guidelines Related to The Development of Protocols for the Appropriate Use and Monitoring of Psychotropic Medication

In the past decade, a variety of practice guidelines have been developed related to the use of psychotropic medication for foster children, including those developed to guide and inform physician prescription practices. Examples include policy statements and guidelines developed by the American Academy of Child and Adolescent Psychiatry (AACAP)[33], the American Academy of Pediatrics,[34] and prescription parameters developed by the State of Texas[35] (later refined by Crismon and Argo, 2009).[36] These efforts are particularly important given that the majority of physicians responsible for prescribing psychotropic medication to foster children are pediatricians or general psychiatrists without formal training in child and adolescent psychiatry and may not have an abundance of exposure to concerns specific to children in foster care.

Perhaps more directly applicable to title IV-B agencies seeking to improve their monitoring and oversight practices of psychotropic medications are two published guidelines that specifically describe components of comprehensive oversight and management plans for children in child welfare. These include an AACAP position statement [37] and guidelines developed by an expert panel convened by the Reach Institute.[38] In addition, a 2010 survey of State written policies and guidelines related to the oversight of psychotropic medication in foster children identified 10 key components of State oversight protocols,[39] and a study by Naylor, et al. (2007) provides additional considerations concerning consent, oversight and policy issues. [40]

Consistent elements found in more than one set of guidelines cited above include the need for written policies to contain provisions for:

- Comprehensive and coordinated screening, assessment, and treatment planning mechanisms to identify children's mental health and trauma-treatment needs (including a psychiatric evaluation, as necessary, to identify needs for psychotropic medication);

- Informed and shared decision-making (consent and assent) and methods for on-going communication between the prescriber, the child, his/her caregivers, other healthcare providers, the child welfare worker, and other key stakeholders;

- Effective medication monitoring at both the client and agency level;

- Availability of mental health expertise and consultation regarding both consent and monitoring issues by a board-certified or board-eligible Child and Adolescent Psychiatrist (at both the agency and individual case level); and

- Mechanisms for accessing and sharing accurate and up-to-date information and educational materials related to mental health and trauma-related interventions (including information about psychotropics) to clinicians, child welfare staff, and consumers.

A particularly helpful aspect of the AACAP guidelines is the categorization of standards in these areas as Minimal, Recommended, and Ideal – features title IV-B agencies may find helpful as they seek to make decisions about improving their current oversight procedures. This approach to categorization of State practices was used in the recent six-state study by GAO of psychotropic medication use by children in foster care to grade each state monitoring system against AACAP recommendations.

In addition, the AACAP guidelines are based on a core set of clinical practice principals specific to psychiatric and pharmacologic treatment of children in foster care. While many professional organizations have practice standards and guidelines related to work with children involved with child welfare (e.g., National Association of Social Workers (NASW) Standards for Social Work Practice in Child Welfare, the Child Welfare League of America's Standards of Excellence, and the Guiding Principles of Systems of Care), the AACAP guidelines are unique in their application to clinical management of psychotropic medications and may be particularly relevant to States, and Tribes when developing the psychotropic medication oversight and monitoring component of their title IV-B plan.

Each title IV-B agency and its service delivery array is unique, making it impractical and inappropriate for every oversight and monitoring plan to be the same. Factors that may influence how States go about developing their plans may include differences in whether the State is largely urban or rural; whether the child welfare service delivery structure is State- or county-administered; the type of Medicaid reimbursement program in place; the availability of qualified practitioners; the availability of automated information systems; and workforce-related issues. As such, each State will need to carefully assess existing oversight mechanisms and evaluate the options in light of how they fit with its own set of needs and challenges. Similarly, Tribes will need to assess the availability of services and qualified practitioners in their service areas to develop monitoring and oversight protocols appropriate to their unique situations.

It should be highlighted that the development of a comprehensive approach to psychotropic medication oversight requires high levels of collaboration among child welfare agencies, professionals, organizations providing foster care and mental health services, children who are recipients of child welfare services, and their families. Nonetheless, most States that responded to the survey described in the 2010 study by Leslie, et. al, acknowledged significant obstacles to collaboration that made it more difficult to develop feasible and sustainable medication oversight plans. Because title

IV-B and Medicaid agencies, pediatricians, and other key health and child welfare experts will need to coordinate in ways they may not have done before, it will also be important to intentionally craft mechanisms to actively engage and involve a broad range of stakeholders.

Federal Initiatives to Encourage the Appropriate Use of Psychotropic Medication

Because children in foster care are typically involved with multiple service delivery systems, including education, health, mental health, Medicaid, and others, a coordinated, multi-system approach is necessary to meaningfully improve outcomes for this population. The Department of Health and Human Services (HHS) is working to facilitate cross-system collaborations for the purposes of promoting improved behavioral health diagnosis, treatment, service delivery and service tracking for children in foster care.

Toward this goal, HHS has identified concrete actions in two areas: (1) increasing oversight and monitoring of psychotropic medications; and (2) expanding the use of evidence-based screening, diagnosis, and treatment of social-emotional, behavioral, and mental health issues among children who have experienced abuse or neglect. Below is a partial list of activities to be undertaken addressing the use of psychotropic medication among children in foster care.

Increased oversight and monitoring: Across the nation, practices related to the oversight and monitoring of psychotropic medications for foster children vary widely, and experts agree that greater controls are needed to ensure safe and appropriate use of psychotropic medications. HHS efforts include the development of a comprehensive Departmental plan focused on ensuring the safe, appropriate, and effective prescription and use of psychotropic therapies for children, and on assisting States and Tribes in strengthening oversight and monitoring practices related to psychotropic medication use among children in foster care. These activities are responsive to recent legislation that requires greater oversight of psychotropic medication use for foster children, and they address long-standing criticisms that State and Federal efforts have failed to adequately regulate psychotropic use in this population.[41]

To help States with the development of the psychotropic medication oversight and monitoring components of their health care oversight and coordination plan, the Administration on Children, Youth and Families (ACYF) is providing multiple opportunities for information-sharing and technical assistance (TA) in advance of the submission of the APSR due June 30, 2012. The TA activities described here primarily focus on State title IV-B agencies, although many may be useful to Tribes, as well. Additional activities directed toward the specific needs of Tribes that administer title IV-B, subpart 1 programs are currently under development.

ACYF technical assistance efforts include:

- A three-part topical webinar series providing additional in-depth information on this topic was produced with assistance from Georgetown University and the American Institutes for Research through an inter-agency agreement with the Substance Abuse and Mental Health Services Administration (SAMHSA). Links to the recordings of these webinars are available on the Child Welfare Information Gateway.

- Additional information, resources, and tools pertaining to the use and oversight of psychotropic medications have been added to the Child Welfare Information Gateway, which will continue to be updated. This includes dissemination of guidelines developed by professional associations and information about exemplary practices in place in some States. One particularly useful document available on the Child Welfare Information Gateway is the Appendix from the 2010 study by Leslie, et. al (referred to above), which references numerous publications and web-based resources on this topic and also highlights useful and innovative tools developed by the States surveyed – many of which may be applicable to States as they refine their own oversight and monitoring procedures.

- Three peer-to-peer learning exchanges to allow information and resource sharing and opportunities to highlight exemplary practices from around the country. These events are designed to provide support to those leaders in child welfare, mental health and Medicaid who are working together to develop the protocols for the oversight and monitoring of psychotropic medications in the health care coordination and oversight component of the title IV-B plan, and will feature brief expert presentations on key considerations related to oversight and monitoring plan components, followed by an open information-sharing dialogue among participants with opportunities to consult with experts in the field.

In additional to this IM which defines the problem and provides resources for States to consider when determining how they will meet the new requirements of the title IV-B plan, CB has issued related Program Instructions ACYF-CB-PI-12-05 and ACYF-CB-PI-12-06that provides further guidance on required APSR content for States and Tribes, respectively.

Finally, after the 2012 APSR submission, ACYF, in collaboration with SAMHSA and the Center for Medicare & Medicaid Services (CMS), is convening a two-day meeting to bring together representatives from State child welfare, Medicaid, and mental health authorities from all fifty States, the District of Columbia, and Puerto Rico to work together to strengthen oversight and monitoring of psychotropic medications for children in foster care.

This meeting entitled, "Because Minds Matter: Collaborating to Strengthen Management of Psychotropic Medication Use for Children and Youth in Foster Care," will be held in August, 2012 to:

- Provide an opportunity for State leaders to enhance existing cross-system efforts to ensure appropriate use of psychotropic medications;

- Showcase collaborative projects and initiatives at State- and local-levels;

- Offer state-of-the-art information on cross-system approaches for improving mental health and well-being outcomes for children and their families;

- Allow participants to strategize to address the mental health and trauma-related needs of children in foster care with evidence-based and evidence-informed interventions; and

- Facilitate each State's development of action steps to improve upon and implement their existing health care oversight and coordination plans.

Additional ongoing activities will also enhance psychotropic medication oversight. CMS is responsible for administering Medicaid funding for health care services for all Medicaid-eligible children, including children in foster care. CMS will continue to share information, establish quality measures, and improve continuity of eligibility and care.[42] They are also working with States to enhance their Drug Utilization Review programs, which allow States to monitor dispensing at the point-of-sale, the pharmacy counter, and to influence prescriber behavior. CMS also will encourage providers to adopt, implement, upgrade, and meaningfully use Electronic Health Records (EHRs) in order to access the Medicaid and Medicare EHR incentive payments. EHRs can improve the consistency and quality of health services for children, especially those whose residences change frequently. The development of quality health homes, standards for behavioral health, and behavioral health coverage for children and adults are among the practices that CMS will promote.

Promoting the increased use of evidence-based screening, assessment, and treatment: Other HHS actions will serve to expand the use of evidence-based and evidence-informed practices for the identification and treatment of social-emotional, behavioral, and mental health problems among children who have experienced maltreatment. There are effective treatments for the mental health disorders and trauma symptoms common among children in foster care. Any effort to ensure the appropriate use of psychotropic medications for these children must be accompanied by increased availability of evidence-based psychosocial treatments that meet the complex needs of children who have experienced maltreatment. Increased access to timely and effective screening, assessment, and non-pharmaceutical treatment will reduce the potential for over-reliance on psychotropic medication as a first-line treatment strategy, and increase the likelihood that children in foster care will exit to positive, permanent settings, with the skills and resources they need to be successful in life. Toward that end, HHS is actively disseminating existing information about effective pharmacological and behavioral practices for children in foster care through webinars and the Child Welfare Information Gateway.[43]

HHS is expanding the evidence base by funding research and demonstration projects that investigate both client-level interventions and system strategies to improve well-being outcomes for children and families. The Agency for Healthcare Research and Quality has contracted for an evidence review of interventions that address child exposure to familial trauma in the form of maltreatment or family violence. 44 Additionally, through its work with the National Child Traumatic Stress Network, SAMHSA continues its work to define best practices and to develop resources to meet the needs of trauma-exposed children and their families. Meanwhile, ACYF has organized its discretionary funding to promote the social and emotional well-being of children and youth who have experienced maltreatment. For example, in FY 2011, a cluster of five grantees received a total of $3.2 million to implement evidence-based, trauma-focused practices and to evaluate their impact on safety, permanency, and well-being outcomes.

Finally, a forthcoming IM on Promoting Social and Emotional Well-Being for Children and Youth Receiving Child Welfare Services will provide States,

Territories and Tribes with more information on the effects of childhood trauma and ways to promote social and emotional wellbeing.

Effective Date: Upon issuance.

Inquiries: Children's Bureau CB Regional Program Managers.

/ s /

Bryan Samuels
Commissioner

ATTACHMENT A: CB REGIONAL OFFICE PROGRAM MANAGERS

I	Region I - Boston Bob Cavanaugh bob.cavanaugh@acf.hhs.gov JFK Federal Building, Rm. 2000 Boston, MA 02203 (617) 565-1020 States: Connecticut, Maine, Massachusetts, New Hampshire, Rhode Island, Vermont	VI	Region VI - Dallas Janis Brown janis.Brown@acf.hhs.gov 1301 Young Street, Suite 945 Dallas, TX 75202-5433 (214) 767-8466 States: Arkansas, Louisiana, New Mexico, Oklahoma, Texas
II	Region II - New York City Junius Scott junius.scott@acf.hhs.gov 26 Federal Plaza, Rm. 4114 New York, NY 10278 (212) 264-2890 States and Territories: New Jersey, New York, Puerto Rico, Virgin Islands	VII	Region VII - Kansas City Rosalyn Wilson rosalyn.wilson@acf.hhs.gov Federal Office Building Room 276 601 E 12th Street Kansas City, MO 64106 (816) 426-3981 States: Iowa, Kansas, Missouri, Nebraska
III	Region III - Philadelphia Lisa Pearson lisa.pearson@acf.hhs.gov 150 S. Independence Mall West - Suite 864 Philadelphia, PA 19106-3499 (215) 861-4000 States: Delaware, District of Columbia, Maryland, Pennsylvania, Virginia, West Virginia	VIII	Region VIII - Denver Marilyn Kennerson marilyn.kennerson@acf.hhs.gov Federal Office Building 1961 Stout Street - 9th Floor Denver, CO 80294-3538 (303) 844-3100 States: Colorado, Montana, North Dakota, South Dakota, Utah, Wyoming

IV	Region IV - Atlanta Ruth Walker ruth.walker@acf.hhs.gov	IX	Region IX - San Francisco Douglas Southard douglas.southard@acf.hhs.gov
	Atlanta Federal Center 61 Forsyth Street S.W. Suite 4M60 Atlanta, GA 30303 (404) 562-2900 States: Alabama, Mississippi, Florida, North Carolina, Georgia, South Carolina, Kentucky, Tennessee		90 7th Street - 9th Floor San Francisco, CA 94103 (415) 437-8425 States and Territories: Arizona, California, Hawaii, Nevada, Outer Pacific—American Samoa Commonwealth of the Northern Marianas, Federated States of Micronesia (Chuuk, Pohnpei, Yap) Guam, Marshall Islands, Palau
V	Region V - Chicago Angela Green angela.green@acf.hhs.gov	X	Region X - Seattle Tina Minor tina.minor@acf.hhs.gov
	233 N. Michigan Avenue Suite 400 Chicago, IL 60601 (312) 353-9672 States: Illinois, Indiana, Michigan, Minnesota, Ohio, Wisconsin		2201 Sixth Avenue, Suite 300, MS-70 Seattle, WA 98121 (206) 615-3657 States: Alaska, Idaho, Oregon, Washington
	Region I - Boston Bob Cavanaugh bob.cavanaugh@acf.hhs.gov		Region VI - Dallas Janis Brown janis.Brown@acf.hhs.gov
	JFK Federal Building, Rm. 2000 Boston, MA 02203 (617) 565-1020 States: Connecticut, Maine, Massachusetts, New Hampshire, Rhode Island, Vermont		1301 Young Street, Suite 945 Dallas, TX 75202-5433 (214) 767-8466 States: Arkansas, Louisiana, New Mexico, Oklahoma, Texas
	Region II - New York City Junius Scott junius.scott@acf.hhs.gov		Region VII - Kansas City Rosalyn Wilson rosalyn.wilson@acf.hhs.gov
	26 Federal Plaza, Rm. 4114 New York, NY 10278 (212) 264-2890 States and Territories: New Jersey, New York, Puerto Rico, Virgin Islands		Federal Office Building Room 276 601 E 12th Street Kansas City, MO 64106 (816) 426-3981 States: Iowa, Kansas, Missouri, Nebraska
	Region III - Philadelphia Lisa Pearson lisa.pearson@acf.hhs.gov		Region VIII - Denver Marilyn Kennerson marilyn.kennerson@acf.hhs.gov

(Continued)

150 S. Independence Mall West - Suite 864 Philadelphia, PA 19106-3499 (215) 861-4000 States: Delaware, District of Columbia, Maryland, Pennsylvania, Virginia, West Virginia	Federal Office Building 1961 Stout Street - 9th Floor Denver, CO 80294-3538 (303) 844-3100 States: Colorado, Montana, North Dakota, South Dakota, Utah, Wyoming
Region IV - Atlanta Ruth Walker ruth.walker@acf.hhs.gov	Region IX - San Francisco Douglas Southard douglas.southard@acf.hhs.gov
Atlanta Federal Center 61 Forsyth Street S.W. Suite 4M60 Atlanta, GA 30303 (404) 562-2900 States: Alabama, Mississippi, Florida, North Carolina, Georgia, South Carolina, Kentucky, Tennessee	90 7th Street - 9th Floor San Francisco, CA 94103 (415) 437-8425 States and Territories: Arizona, California, Hawaii, Nevada, Outer Pacific—American Samoa Commonwealth of the Northern Marianas, Federated States of Micronesia (Chuuk, Pohnpei, Yap) Guam, Marshall Islands, Palau
Region V - Chicago Angela Green angela.green@acf.hhs.gov	Region X - Seattle Tina Minor tina.minor@acf.hhs.gov
233 N. Michigan Avenue Suite 400 Chicago, IL 60601 (312) 353-9672 States: Illinois, Indiana, Michigan, Minnesota, Ohio, Wisconsin	2201 Sixth Avenue, Suite 300, MS-70 Seattle, WA 98121 (206) 615-3657 States: Alaska, Idaho, Oregon, Washington

End Notes

[1] Some Tribes receiving title IV-B funding do not directly operate foster care programs. In these instances, the State agency is responsible for providing foster care services for Tribal children needing such services and for developing the health care oversight and coordination plan.

[2] Zito, J.M., Safer, D.J, dosReis, S., Gardner, J.F., Bole, M. & Lynch, F. (2000). Trends in the prescribing of psychotropic medications to preschoolers. JAMA, 238(8), 1025-1030.

[3] ZitoJ M, Safer DJ, Sai D et al. (2008). Psychotropic medication patterns among youth in foster care. Pediatrics, 121:e157-e163.

[4] dosReis, S., Zito, J.M., Safer, D.J., Soeken, K.L. (2001). Mental Health Services for Foster Care and Disabled Youth. American Journal of Public Health, 91(7), 1094-1099.

[5] McMillen JC, Fedoravicius N, Rowe J, Zima BT, Ware N. (2007) A crisis of credibility: Professionals' concerns about the psychiatric care provided to clients of the child welfare system. Administration & Policy in Mental Health and Mental Health Services Research, 34:203-12.

[6] Office of the Texas Comptroller. (2007) Texas Health Care Claims Study: Special Report on Foster Children. Texas Comptroller of Public Accounts.

[7] Olfson, M, Marcus, S.C., Weissman, M.M., & Jensen, P.S. (2002). National trends in the use of psychotropic medications by children. Journal of American Child and Adolescent Psychiatry, 41(5), 514-521.

[8] Leslie, LK; Raghavan, R; Zhang, J; & Aarons, GA. (2010). Rates of psychotropic medication use over time among youth in child welfare/child protective services. Journal of Child and Adolescent Psychopharmacology. 20(2):135.

[9] Zima, B. T., Hurlburt, M. S., Knapp, P., Ladd, H., Tang, L., Duan, N. et al. (2005). Quality of publicly-funded outpatient specialty mental health care for common childhood psychiatric disorders in California. Journal of the American Academy of Child Adolescent Psychiatry, 44(2), 130-144.

[10] Ferguson, D.G, Glesener, D.C. & Raschick, M. (2006). Psychotropic Drug Use with European American and American Indian Children in Foster Care. Journal of Child and Adolescent Psychopharmacology, 16(4), 474-481.

[11] Raghavan, R; Zima, BT; Anderson, RM; Leibowitz, AA; Schuster, MA; & Landsverk, J. (2005). Psychotropic medication use in a national probability sample of children in the child welfare system. Journal of child and adolescent psychopharmacology. 15(1):97.

[12] Raghavan, R; Gyanesh, L; Kohl, P; & Hamilton, B. (2010). Interstate variations in psychotropic medication use among a national sample of children in the child welfare system. Child Maltreatment. 15(2): 121-131.

[13] Leslie, L K., Raghavan, R, Hurley, M, Zhang, J, Landsverk, J, Aarons, G. (2011) Investigating geographic variation in use of psychotropic medications among youth in child welfare. Child Abuse & Neglect, 35(5):333-42.

[14] Zima, B.T., Bussing, R., Crecelius, G.M., Kaufman, A. & Belin, T.R. (1999) Psychotropic medication use among children in foster care: Relationship to severe psychiatric disorders. American Journal of Public Health, 889(11), 1732-1735.

[15] The National Survey of Child and Adolescent Well-Being (NSCAW) is a longitudinal study required by the Personal Responsibility and Work Opportunity Reconciliation Act of 1996 overseen by the Administration on Children and Families. It is a key source of information about the social and emotional well-being of children who have experienced maltreatment, including information on rates of psychotropic medication use.

[16] White, CR; Havalchak, A; Jackson, L; O'Brien, K; & Pecora, PJ. (2007). Mental Health, Ethnicity, Sexuality, and Spirituality among Youth in Foster Care: Findings from The Casey Field Office Mental Health Study. Casey Family Programs.

[17] Griffin, G; McClelland, Holzberg, M; Stolbach, B; Maj, N; & Kisiel, C (In Press). Addressing the impact of trauma before diagnosing mental illness in child welfare. Child Welfare.

[18] Center for Health Care Strategies, Inc. (Forthcoming). Analysis of Medicaid Claims Data for 2005.

[19] Jensen, P.S., Bhatara, V.S., Vitiello, B., Hoagwood, K., Feil, M., & Burke, L.B. (1999). Psychoactive Medication Prescribing Practices for U.S. Children: Gaps Between Research

and Clinical Practice. Journal of the American Academy of Child & Adolescent Psychiatry, 38(5), 557-565.

[20] Wethington, H.R., Hahn, R.A., Fuqua-Whitley, D.S., Sipe, T.A., Crosby, A.E., Johnson, R.L., Liberman, A.M., Mos´cicki, E., Price, L.N., Tuma, F.K., Kalra, G., Chattopadhyay, S.K, & Task Force on Community Preventive Services. (2008). The Effectiveness of Interventions to Reduce Psychological Harm from Traumatic Events Among Children and Adolescents: A Systematic Review. American Journal of Preventative Medicine, 35(3), 287–313.

[21] Olfson, M, Marcus, S.C., Weissman, M.M., & Jensen, P.S. (2002). National trends in the use of psychotropic medications by children. Journal of American Child and Adolescent Psychiatry, 41(5), 514-521.

[22] Zito, JM; et al., (2008). Psychotropic medication patterns among youth in foster care. Pediatrics. 121(1): e157.

[23] Roberts R., Rodriguez W., Murphy D., and Crescenzi T.(2003). Pediatric drug labeling. JAMA, 290, 905- 911.

[24] FDA regulations allow prescription of approved medications for other than their approved indications.

[25] Retrieved from: http://www.dshs.state.tx.us/mhprograms/pdf/PsychotropicMedication UtilizationParameters FosterChildren.pdf).

[26] Naylor, M.W., Davidson, C., Ortega-Piron, D.J., Bass, A., Guitierrez, A, Hall, A. (2007). Psychotropic medication management for youths in state care: Pharmacoepidemiology and policy considerations. Child Welfare, 86(5):175- 192.

[27] Zito, J.M., Derivan, A.T., Kratochvil, C.J., Safer, D.J., Fegert, J.M., & Greenhill, L.L. (2008), Child and Adolescent Psychiatry and Mental Health. Off-label psychopharmacologic prescribing for children: History supports close clinical monitoring.

[28] Zito, J.M., Safer, D.J, dosReis, S., Gardner, J.F., Bole, M. & Lynch, F. (2000). Trends in the prescribing of psychotropic medications to preschoolers. JAMA, 238(8), 1025-1030.

[29] U.S. Government Accountability Office. Foster Children: HHS Guidance Could Help States Improve Oversight of Psychotropic Prescriptions. Washington, D.C.: General Accountability Office; 2011. GAO-12-201. Retrieved from: http://www.gao.gov/products/ GAO-12-270T.

[30] Gleason M.M., Egger HL, Emslie G.J., Greenhill L.L., Kowatch RA, Lieberman AF, Luby J.L., Owens J, Scahill L.D., Scheering, M.S., Stafford B, Wise B, Zeanah C.H.(2007). Psychopharmacological treatment for very young children: Contexts and guidelines. Journal of the American Academy of Child and Adolescent Psychiatry, 46(12):1532-1572.

[31] Crystal, S; Olfson, M; Huang, C; Pincus, H; & Gerhard, T. (2009). Broadened use of atypical antipsychotics: Safety, effectiveness, and policy challenges. Health Affairs, 28(5):770. (http://content.healthaffairs.org/content/28/5/w770.full.html).

[32] Mackie, T.I., Hyde, J., Rodday, A.M., Dawson, E., Lakshmikanthan, R., Bellonci, C., Schoonover, D.R., and Leslie, L.K. (2011). Psychotropic medication oversight for youth in foster care: A national perspective on state child welfare policy and practice guidelines. Child and Youth Services Review, 33, 2213-2220.

[33] American Academy of Child and Adolescent Psychiatry. The Mental Health Needs of Children in Foster Care, Policies and Best Principles. AACAP website; http://www.aacap.org.

[34] American Academy of Pediatrics. (2002). Health care of young children in foster care. Pediatrics, 109, 536-541.

[35] Texas Department of State Health Services (2007). Psychotropic medication utilization parameters for foster children. Retrieved from http://dshs.state.tx.us/mhprograms/ pdf/Psychotropic MedicationUtilizationParametersFosterChildren.pdf.

[36] Crismon, M.L., & Argo, T. (2009). The use of psychotropic medication for children in foster care. Child Welfare, 88, 71-100.

[37] AACAP Position Statement on Oversight of Psychotropic Use for Children in State Custody: A Best Principles Guideline. AACAP website only. http://www.aacap.org/galleries/PracticeInformation/FosterCare_BestPrinciples_FINAL.pdf.

[38] Romanelli, L.H., Landsverk, J., Levitt, J.M., Leslie, L.K., Hurley, M.M., Bellonci, C. et al. (2009). Best practices for mental health in child welfare: Screening, assessment, and treatment guidelines. Child Welfare, 88(1), 163-188.

[39] Leslie, L.K., Mackie, T., Dawson, E.H., Bellonci, C., Schoonover, D.R., Rodday, A.M., et al. (2010). Multi-state study on psychotropic medication oversight in foster care. Boston, MA: Tufts Clinical Translational Science Institute.

[40] Naylor, M., Davidson, C., Ortega-Piron, D., Bass, A, Guitierrez, A., and Hall, A. (2007). Psychotropic medication management for youth in state care: Consent, oversight, and policy considerations. Child Welfare, 86(5), 175.

[41] Camp, A.R. (2011). A mistreated epidemic: State and federal failure to adequately regulate psychotropic medications prescribed to children in foster care. Temple Law Review. Retrieved from http://ssrn.com/abstract=1567682.

[42] Retrieved from: http://www.childwelfare.gov/systemwide/mentalhealth/ effectiveness/jointlettermeds.pdf.

[43] The Child Welfare Information Gateway can be accessed through the following website: http://www.childwelfare.gov/. Child Welfare Information Gateway connects child welfare and other professionals to information and resources related to protecting children and strengthening families.

[44] Retrieved from: http://www.effectivehealthcare.ahrq.gov/index.cfm/search-for-guides-reviews-andreports/?pageaction=displayproduct&productid=846.

INDEX

O

officials, 17, 68, 70, 71, 73, 74, 89, 90, 91, 92, 93, 94, 95, 96, 97, 98, 99, 100, 101, 102, 104, 106, 107, 108
Oklahoma, 51, 126, 127
olanzapine, 83
opportunities, 23, 97, 119, 122, 123
outpatient, 8, 9, 10, 57, 86, 100, 119, 129
oversight, vii, 2, 3, 18, 19, 20, 21, 22, 23, 25, 26, 27, 28, 29, 32, 33, 34, 35, 36, 38, 39, 53, 63, 68, 70, 72, 74, 76, 86, 89, 90, 92, 93, 94, 95, 96, 99, 100, 101, 102, 108, 110, 111, 118, 119, 120, 121, 122, 123, 124, 128, 130, 131

P

paranoia, 81
parental consent, 44
parents, vii, 1, 4, 8, 11, 13, 15, 19, 20, 31, 37, 46, 47, 52, 54, 75, 94, 98
participants, 17, 55, 100, 123, 124
pediatrician, 46, 79
personality disorder, 81
pharmaceutical, 8, 16, 17, 125
pharmacological treatment, 118
pharmacotherapy, 60
Philadelphia, 57, 126, 127, 128
physical abuse, 80, 81, 84
physicians, 18, 27, 46, 52, 88, 118, 120
policy, 3, 4, 25, 27, 29, 32, 39, 51, 53, 63, 92, 119, 120, 130, 131
policy issues, 3, 32, 120
population, 5, 6, 17, 34, 35, 55, 57, 68, 72, 76, 102, 106, 111, 112, 113, 116, 118, 122
post-traumatic stress disorder (PTSD), 68, 81, 114, 115
preschool children, 118
preschoolers, 118, 128, 130
prescription drugs, 7, 24, 35
principles, 61, 72, 92
private practice, 57

psychiatric diagnosis, 86
psychiatric disorders, 129
psychiatrist, 2, 29, 31, 36, 46, 48, 50, 51, 79, 92, 93, 99, 104
psychiatry, 6, 30, 46, 50, 51, 56, 73, 74, 103, 104, 120
psychological assessments, 69
psychopharmacological treatments, 115
psychopharmacology, 61, 129
psychosis, 81, 119
psychosocial functioning, 80
psychosocial interventions, 4, 20, 21, 24, 108
psychotherapy, 80, 91
psychotropic drugs, 10, 14, 16, 54, 57, 68, 69, 93, 107, 116, 118
psychotropic medications, vii, 1, 2, 3, 4, 8, 10, 11, 12, 14, 16, 17, 19, 20, 21, 22, 25, 26, 27, 30, 31, 32, 33, 34, 35, 36, 38, 39, 41, 44, 45, 46, 50, 51, 52, 53, 54, 61, 63, 68, 69, 70, 71, 72, 73, 74, 75, 76, 83, 84, 86, 87, 88, 89, 90, 92, 93, 94, 95, 96, 97, 99, 100, 101, 102, 103, 108, 109, 110, 111, 112, 114, 115, 116, 117, 118, 119, 120, 121, 122, 123, 124, 125, 128, 129, 130, 131
public health, 42, 119
Puerto Rico, 124, 126, 127

Q

quality assurance, 52
quetiapine, 83, 84

R

recommendations, iv, 16, 19, 25, 83, 86, 117, 118, 121
reform(s), 32 63
regulations, 19, 62, 74, 130
relatives, 4, 11
requirement(s), 4, 7, 18, 20, 21, 23, 25, 27, 51, 59, 60, 62, 96, 102, 103, 106, 107, 109, 110, 111, 124

S

T

V

W

Washington, 45, 104, 106, 108, 127, 128, 130
weight gain, 17
welfare, 2, 3, 4, 7, 8, 9, 10, 11, 12, 13, 17, 18, 19, 20, 21, 22, 23, 24, 26, 27, 28, 30, 31, 33, 35, 36, 41, 42, 43, 44, 45, 46, 47, 48, 49, 50, 51, 52, 53, 54, 55, 58, 61, 62, 64, 68, 71, 73, 74, 75, 76, 89, 90, 91, 92, 94, 96, 97, 98, 99, 100, 101, 102, 103, 107, 108, 110, 111, 112, 113, 114, 120, 121, 123, 124, 129, 130, 131
welfare law, 3, 27
welfare system, 10, 11, 12, 76, 98, 112, 114, 129
well-being, 4, 18, 20, 22, 24, 27, 124, 125
well-being outcomes, 24, 124, 125

Y

young people, 35, 112